Anti-Inflammatory Cookbook for the Hardened Meat-Eaters

Mouthwatering Recipes To Reduce Inflammation in the Body by Cooking Delicious Red Meat

By
Olga Jones

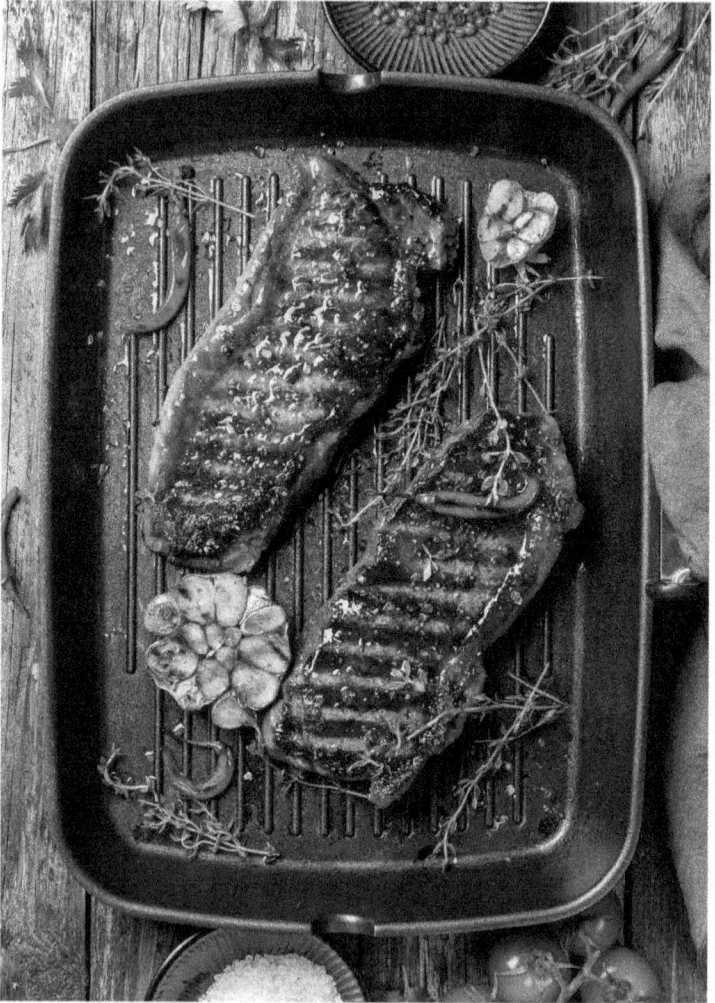

Table of Contents

INTRODUCTION

What is the Anti-Inflammatory Diet?

The anti-inflammatory diet is the best choice for your health if you have conditions that cause inflammation. Such conditions are asthma, chronic peptic ulcer, tuberculosis, rheumatoid arthritis, periodontitis, Crohn's disease, sinusitis, active hepatitis, etc. Along with medical treatment, proper nutrition is very important. An anti-inflammatory diet can help to reduce the pain from inflammation for a few notches. Such a diet isn't a panacea but a significant help in any treatment. Inflammation is a natural response of your body to infections, injuries, and illnesses. The classic symptoms of inflammation are redness, pain, heat, and swelling. Nevertheless, some diseases don't have any symptoms. Such illnesses are diabetes, heart disease, cancer, etc. That's why we should care about our health permanently and an anti-inflammatory diet is one of the ways for it.

Inflammation is your immune system's response to injury or unwanted microbes in your body. It is a natural process and vital part of your body's healing process. When inflammation becomes systemic and chronic, however, it becomes a problem, and measures need to be taken. This type of inflammation serves no purpose, and can cause a lot of harm to the body.

This book has a LOT of recipes, and not every recipe might work for you. For example, if you're allergic to dairy or gluten, the recipes containing those ingredients will cause more harm than good. However, substitutions are possible for all of these, so you will be fine following this book as long as you keep an eye on the ingredients and use a bit of creativity where you have to! Once you understand the fundamentals of the diet, you will be fully equipped to create your own recipes from scratch!This is the most important information that you should know before starting a diet. Any diet is not a magic remedy for all diseases; it is a support for the body during a difficult time of treatment. Start your new healthy life from one small step and you will see the huge results within half a year. You can be sure that your body will be thankful to you by giving you a fresh look and energy for new achievements.

Ground Lamb with Peas

Yield: 4 servings
Preparation Time: 15 minutes
Cooking Time: 55 minutes

Ingredients:
- 1 tablespoon coconut oil
- 3 dried red chilies
- 1 (2-inch) cinnamon stick
- 3 green cardamom pods
- ½ teaspoon cumin seeds
- 1 medium red onion, chopped
- 1 (¾-inch) piece fresh ginger, minced
- 4 garlic cloves, minced
- 1½ teaspoons ground coriander
- ½ teaspoon garam masala
- ½ teaspoon ground cumin
- ½ teaspoon ground turmeric
- ¼ teaspoon ground nutmeg
- 2 bay leaves
- 1 pound lean ground lamb
- ½ cup Roma tomatoes, chopped
- 1-1½ cups water
- 1 cup fresh green peas, shelled
- 2 tablespoons plain Greek yogurt, whipped
- ¼ cup fresh cilantro, chopped
- Salt and freshly ground black pepper, to taste

Directions:
1. In a Dutch oven, melt coconut oil medium-high heat.
2. Add red chilies, cinnamon stick, cardamom pods and cumin seeds and sauté for around thirty seconds.
3. Add onion and sauté for about 3-4 minutes.
4. Add ginger, garlic cloves and spices and sauté for around thirty seconds.
5. Add lamb and cook for approximately 5 minutes.
6. Add tomatoes and cook for approximately 10 min.
7. Stir in water and green peas and cook, covered approximately 25-thirty minutes.
8. Stir in yogurt, cilantro, salt and black pepper and cook for around 4-5 minutes.
9. Serve hot.

Broiled Lamb Shoulder

Yield: 10 servings
Preparation Time: 10 minutes
Cooking Time: 8-10 minutes

Ingredients:
- 2 tablespoons fresh ginger, minced
- 2 tablespoons garlic, minced
- ¼ cup fresh lemongrass stalk, minced
- ¼ cup fresh orange juice
- ¼ cup coconut aminos
- Freshly ground black pepper, to taste
- 2 pound lamb shoulder, trimmed

Directions:
1. In a bowl, mix together all ingredients except lamb shoulder.
2. In a baking dish, squeeze lamb shoulder and coat the lamb with half in the marinade mixture generously.
3. Reserve remaining mixture.
4. Refrigerate to marinate for overnight.
5. Preheat the broiler of oven. Place a rack inside a broiler pan about 4-5-inches from heating unit.
6. Remove lamb shoulder from refrigerator and remove excess marinade.
7. Broil approximately 4-5 minutes from both sides.
8. Serve with all the reserved marinade like a sauce.

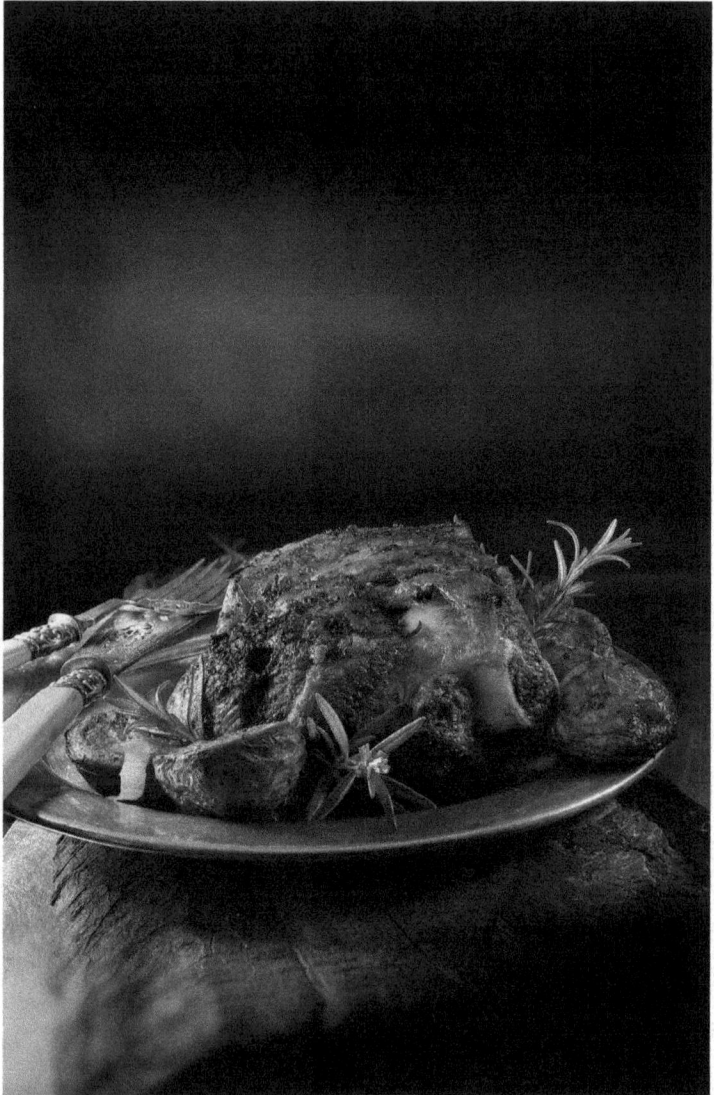

Roasted Lamb Chops

Yield: 4 servings
Preparation Time: 15 minutes
Cooking Time: half an hour

Ingredients:
For Lamb Marinade:
- 4 garlic cloves, chopped
- 1 (2-inch) piece fresh ginger, chopped
- 2 green chilies, seeded and chopped
- 1 teaspoon fresh lime zest
- 2 teaspoons garam masala
- 1 teaspoon ground coriander
- 1 teaspoon ground cumin
- ½ teaspoon ground cinnamon
- 1 teaspoon coconut oil, melted
- 2 tablespoons fresh lime juice
- 6-7 tablespoons plain Greek yogurt
- 1 (8-bone) rack of lamb, trimmed
- 2 onions, sliced

For Relish:
- ½ of garlic herb, chopped
- 1 (1-inch) piece fresh ginger, chopped
- ¼ cup fresh cilantro, chopped
- ¼ cup fresh mint, chopped
- 1 green chili, seeded and chopped
- 1 teaspoon fresh lime zest
- 1 teaspoon organic honey

- 2 tablespoons fresh apple juice
- 2 tablespoons fresh lime juice

Directions:
1. For chops, in a very mixer, add all ingredients except yogurt, chops and onions and pulse till smooth.
2. Transfer the mixture in a large bowl with yogurt and stir to combine well.
3. Add chops and coat with mixture generously.
4. Refrigerate to marinate for approximately twenty four hours.
5. Preheat the oven to 375 degrees F. Line a roasting pan with a foil paper.
6. Place the onion wedges in the bottom of prepared roasting pan.
7. Arrange rack of lamb over onion wedges.
8. Roast approximately half an hour.
9. Meanwhile for relish in the blender, add all ingredients and pulse till smooth.
10. Serve chops and onions alongside relish.

Lamb Burgers with Avocado Dip

Yield: 4-6 servings
Preparation Time: 20 minutes
Cooking Time: 10 minutes

Ingredients:
For Burgers:
- 1 (2-inch) piece fresh ginger, grated
- 1 pound lean ground lamb
- 1 medium onion, grated
- 2 minced garlic cloves
- 1 bunch fresh mint leaves, chopped finely
- 2 teaspoons ground coriander
- 2 teaspoons ground cumin
- ½ teaspoon ground allspice
- ½ teaspoon ground cinnamon
- Salt and freshly ground black pepper, to taste
- 1 tbsp essential olive oil

For Dip:
- 3 small cucumbers, peeled and grated
- 1 avocado, peeled, pitted and chopped
- ½ of garlic oil, crushed
- 2 tablespoons fresh lemon juice
- 2 tablespoons olive oil
- 2 tablespoons fresh dill, chopped finely
- 2 tablespoons chives, chopped finely
- Salt and freshly ground black pepper, to taste

Directions:

1. Preheat the broiler of oven. Lightly, grease a broiler pan.

2. For burgers in a big bowl, squeeze the juice of ginger.

3. Add remaining ingredients and mix till well combined.

4. Make equal sized burgers from your mixture.

5. Arrange the burgers in broiler pan and broil approximately 5 minutes per side.

6. Meanwhile for dip, squeeze the cucumbers juice in a bowl.

7. In a blender, add avocado, garlic, lemon juice and oil and pulse till smooth.

8. Transfer the avocado mixture in a bowl.

9. Add remaining ingredients and stir to mix.

10. Serve the burgers with avocado dip.

Baked Meatballs & Scallions

Yield: 4-6 servings
Preparation Time: 20 min
Cooking Time: 35 minutes

Ingredients:
For Meatballs:

- 1 lemongrass stalk, outer skin peeled and chopped
- 1 (1½-inch) piece fresh ginger, sliced
- 3 garlic cloves, chopped
- 1 cup fresh cilantro leaves, chopped roughly
- ½ cup fresh basil leaves, chopped roughly
- 2 tablespoons plus 1 teaspoon fish sauce
- 2 tablespoons water
- 2 tablespoons fresh lime juice
- ½ pound lean ground pork
- 1 pound lean ground lamb
- 1 carrot, peeled and grated
- 1 organic egg, bea10

For Scallions:

- 16 stalks scallions, trimmed
- 2 tablespoons coconut oil, melted
- Salt, to taste
- ½ cup water

Directions:
1. Preheat the oven to 375 degrees F. Grease a baking dish.

2. In a blender, add lemongrass, ginger, garlic, fresh herbs, fish sauce, water and lime juice and pulse till chopped finely.

3. Transfer the amalgamation in a bowl with remaining ingredients and mix till well combined.

4. Make about 1-inch balls from mixture.

5. Arrange the balls into prepared baking dish in a single layer.

6. In another rimmed baking dish, arrange scallion stalks in a very single layer.

7. Drizzle with coconut oil and sprinkle with salt.

8. Pour water in the baking dish 1nd with a foil paper cover it tightly.

9. Bake the scallion for around a half-hour.

10. Bake the meatballs for approximately 30-35 minutes. Pork with Bell Pepper This stir fry not simply tastes wonderful but additionally is packed with nutritious benefits.

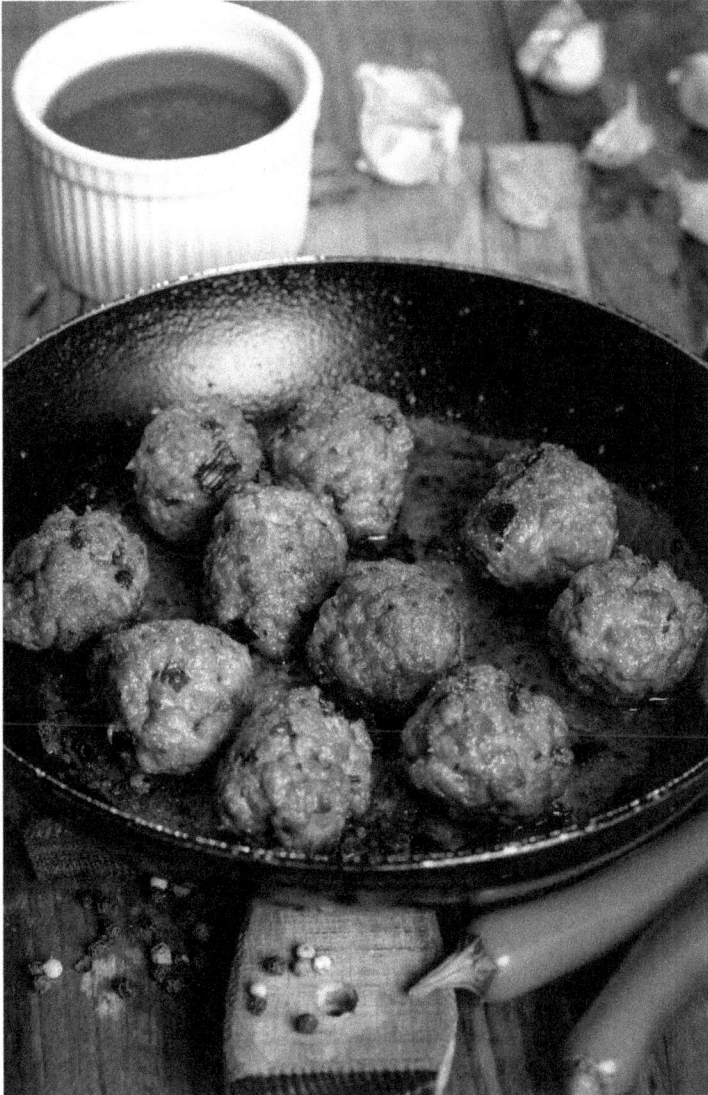

Pork with Pineapple

Yield: 4 servings
Preparation Time: 15 minutes
Cooking Time: 14 minutes

Ingredients:

- 2 tablespoons coconut oil
- 1½ pound pork tenderloin, trimmed and cut into bite sized pieces
- 1 onion, chopped
- 2 minced garlic cloves
- 1 (1-inch) piece fresh ginger, minced
- 20-ounce pineapple, cut into chunks
- 1 large red bell pepper, seeded and chopped
- ¼ cup fresh pineapple juice
- ¼ cup coconut aminos
- Salt and freshly ground black pepper, to taste

Directions:

1. In a substantial skillet, melt coconut oil on high heat.

2. Add pork and stir fry approximately 4-5 minutes.

3. Transfer the pork right into a bowl.

4. In exactly the same skillet, heat remaining oil on medium heat.

5. Add onion, garlic and ginger and sauté for around 2 minutes.

6. Stir in pineapple and bell pepper and stir fry for around 3 minutes.

7. Stir in pork, pineapple juice and coconut aminos and cook for around 3-4 minutes.

8. Serve hot.

Pork Chili

Yield: 8 servings
Preparation Time: quarter-hour
Cooking Time: 60 minutes

Ingredients:
- 2 tablespoons extra-virgin organic olive oil
- 2 pound ground pork
- 1 medium red bell pepper, seeded and chopped
- 1 medium onion, chopped
- 5 garlic cloves, chopped finely
- 1 (2-inch) part of hot pepper, minced
- 1 tablespoon ground cumin
- 1 teaspoon ground turmeric
- 3 tablespoon chili powder
- ½ teaspoon chipotle chili powder
- Salt and freshly ground black pepper, to taste
- 1 cup chicken broth
- 1 (28-ounce) can fire-roasted crushed tomatoes
- 2 medium bok choy heads, sliced
- 1 avocado, peeled, pitted and chopped

Directions:
1. In a sizable pan, heat oil on medium heat.
2. Add pork and stir fry for about 5 minutes.
3. Add bell pepper, onion, garlic, hot pepper and spices and stir fry for
approximately 5 minutes.
4. Add broth and tomatoes and convey with a boil.

5. Stir in bok choy and cook, covered for approximately twenty minutes.

6. Uncover and cook approximately 20-half an hour.

7. Serve hot while using topping of avocado.

Glazed Pork chops with Peach

Yield: 2 servings
Preparation Time: quarter-hour
Cooking Time: 16 minutes

Ingredients:
- 2 boneless pork chops
- Salt and freshly ground black pepper, to taste
- 1 ripe yellow peach, peeled, pitted, chopped and divided
- 1 tbsp organic olive oil
- 2 tablespoons shallot, minced
- 2 tablespoons garlic, minced
- 2 tablespoons fresh ginger, minced
- 1 tablespoon organic honey
- 1 tablespoon balsamic vinegar
- 1 tablespoon coconut aminos
- ¼ teaspoon red pepper flakes, crushed
- ¼ cup water

Directions:
1. Sprinkle the pork chops with salt and black pepper generously.
2. In a blender, add 1 / 2 of peach and pulse till a puree forms.
3. Reserve remaining peach.
4. In a skillet, heat oil on medium heat.
5. Add shallots and sauté approximately 1-2 minutes.
6. Add garlic and ginger and sauté approximately 1 minute.
7. Add remaining ingredients and lower heat to medium-low.

8. Bring to your boil and simmer for approximately 4-5 minutes or till a sticky glaze forms.

9. Remove from heat and reserve 1/3 with the glaze and keep aside.

10. Coat the chops with remaining glaze.

11. Heat a nonstick skillet on medium-high heat.

12. Add chops and sear for around 4 minutes from both sides.

13. Transfer the chops in a plate and coat with all the remaining glaze evenly.

14. Top with reserved chopped peach and serve.

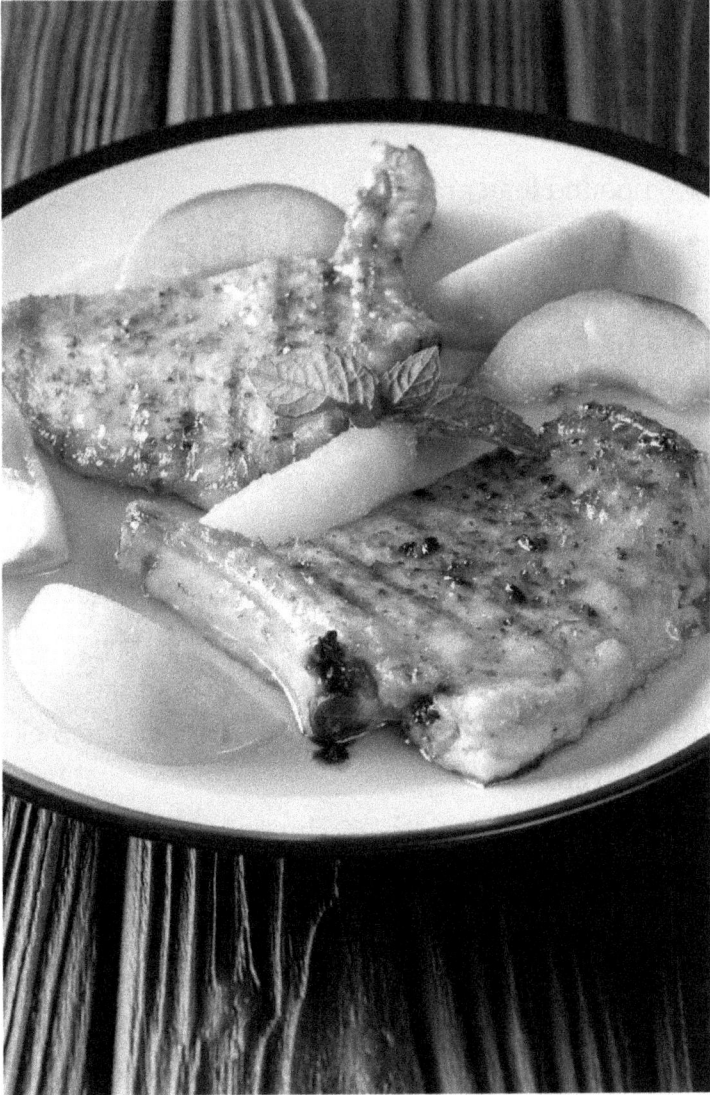

Baked Pork & Mushroom Meatballs

Yield: 6 servings
Preparation Time: 15 minutes
Cooking Time: fifteen minutes

Ingredients:

- 1 pound lean ground pork
- 1 organic egg white, beaten
- 4 fresh shiitake mushrooms, stemmed and minced
- 1 tablespoon fresh parsley, minced
- 1 tablespoon fresh basil leaves, minced
- 1 tablespoon fresh mint leaves, minced
- 2 teaspoons fresh lemon zest, grated finely
- 1½ teaspoons fresh ginger, grated finely
- Salt and freshly ground black pepper, to taste

Directions:

1. Preheat the oven to 425 degrees F. Arrange the rack inside center of oven.

2. Line a baking sheet with parchment paper.

3. In a sizable bowl, add all ingredients and mix till well combined.

4. Make small equal-sized balls from the mixture.

5. Arrange the balls onto prepared baking sheet in a single layer.

6. Bake for approximately 12-quarter-hour or till done completely.

Beef with Carrot & Broccoli

Yield: 4 servings
Preparation Time: fifteen minutes
Cooking Time: 14 minutes

Ingredients:

- 2 tablespoons coconut oil, divided
- 2 medium garlic cloves, minced
- 1 pound beef sirloin steak, trimmed and sliced into thin strips
- Salt, to taste
- ¼ cup chicken broth
- 2 teaspoons fresh ginger, grated
- 1 tablespoon ground flax seeds
- ½ teaspoon red pepper flakes, crushed
- ¼ teaspoon freshly ground black pepper
- 1 large carrot, peeled and sliced thinly
- 2 cups broccoli florets
- 1 medium scallion, sliced thinly

Directions:

1. In a substantial skillet, heat 1 tablespoon of oil on medium-high heat.
2. Add garlic and sauté approximately 1 minute.
3. Add beef and salt and cook for approximately 4-5 minutes or till browned.
4. With a slotted spoon, transfer the beef in a bowl.
5. Remove the liquid from skillet.

6. In a bowl, mix together broth, ginger, flax seeds, red pepper flakes and black pepper.

7. In a similar skillet, heat remaining oil on medium heat.

8. Add carrot, broccoli and ginger mixture and cook for approximately 3-4 minutes or till desired doneness.

9. Stir in beef and scallion and cook for around 3-4 minutes.

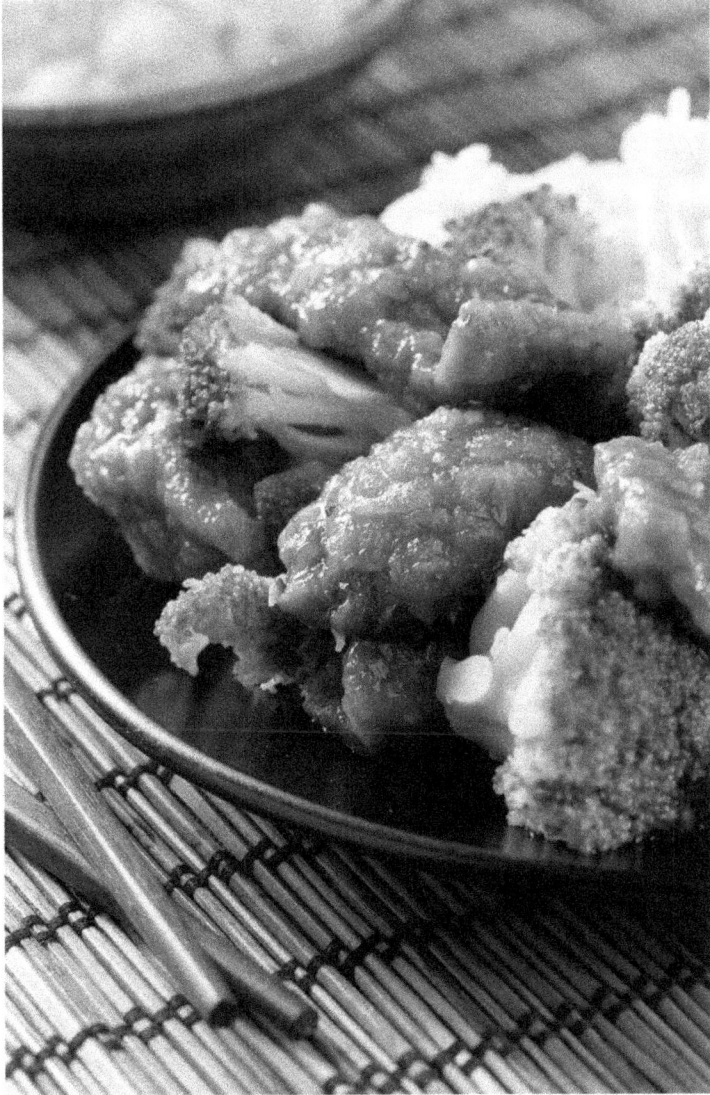

Citrus Beef with Bok Choy

Yield: 4 servings
Preparation Time: fifteen minutes
Cooking Time: 11 minutes

Ingredients:
For Marinade:

- 2 minced garlic cloves
- 1 (1-inch) piece fresh ginger, grated
- 1/3 cup fresh orange juice
- ½ cup coconut aminos
- 2 teaspoons fish sauce
- 2 teaspoons Sriracha
- 1¼ pound sirloin steak, trimmed and sliced thinly

For Veggies:

- 2 tablespoons coconut oil, divided
- 3-4 wide strips of fresh orange zest
- 1 jalapeño pepper, sliced thinly
- ½ pound string beans, stemmed and halved crosswise
- 1 tablespoon arrowroot powder
- ½ pound bok choy, chopped
- 2 teaspoons sesame seeds

Directions:
1. For marinade in a big bowl, mix together garlic, ginger, orange juice, coconut aminos, fish sauce and Sriracha.
2. Add beef and coat with marinade generously.

---

3. Refrigerate to marinate for around a couple of hours.

4. In a substantial skillet, heat oil on medium-high heat.

5. Add orange zest and sauté approximately 2 minutes.

6. Remove beef from bowl, reserving the marinade.

7. In the skillet, add beef and increase the heat to high.

8. Stir fry for about 2-3 minutes or till browned.

9. With a slotted spoon, transfer the beef and orange strips right into a bowl.

10. With a paper towel, wipe out the skillet.

11. In a similar skillet, heat remaining oil on medium-high heat.

12. Add jalapeño pepper and string beans and stir fry for about 3-4 minutes.

13. Meanwhile add arrowroot powder in reserved marinade and stir to mix.

14. In the skillet, add marinade mixture, beef and bok choy and cook for about 1-2 minutes. 15. Serve hot with garnishing of sesame seeds.

Beef with Asparagus & Bell Pepper

Yield: 4-5 servings
Preparation Time: fifteen minutes
Cooking Time: 13 minutes

Ingredients:

- 4 garlic cloves, minced
- 3 tablespoons coconut aminos
- 1/8 teaspoon red pepper flakes, crushed
- 1/8 teaspoon ground ginger
- Freshly ground black pepper, to taste
- 1 bunch asparagus, trimmed and halved
- 2 tablespoons olive oil, divided
- 1 pound flank steak, trimmed and sliced thinly
- 1 red bell pepper, seeded and sliced
- 3 tablespoons water
- 2 teaspoons arrowroot powder

Directions:

1 In a bowl, mix together garlic, coconut aminos, red pepper flakes, crushed, ground ginger and black pepper. Keep aside.

2. In a pan of boiling water, cook asparagus for about 2 minutes.

3. Drain and rinse under cold water.

4. In a substantial skillet, heat 1 tablespoon of oil on medium-high heat.

5. Add beef and stir fry for around 3-4 minutes.

6. With a slotted spoon, transfer the beef in a bowl.

7. In a similar skillet, heat remaining oil on medium heat.

8. Add asparagus and bell pepper and stir fry for approximately 2-3 minutes.

9. Meanwhile in the bowl, mix together water and arrowroot powder.

10. Stir in beef, garlic mixture and arrowroot mixture and cook for around 3-4 minutes or
till desired thickness.

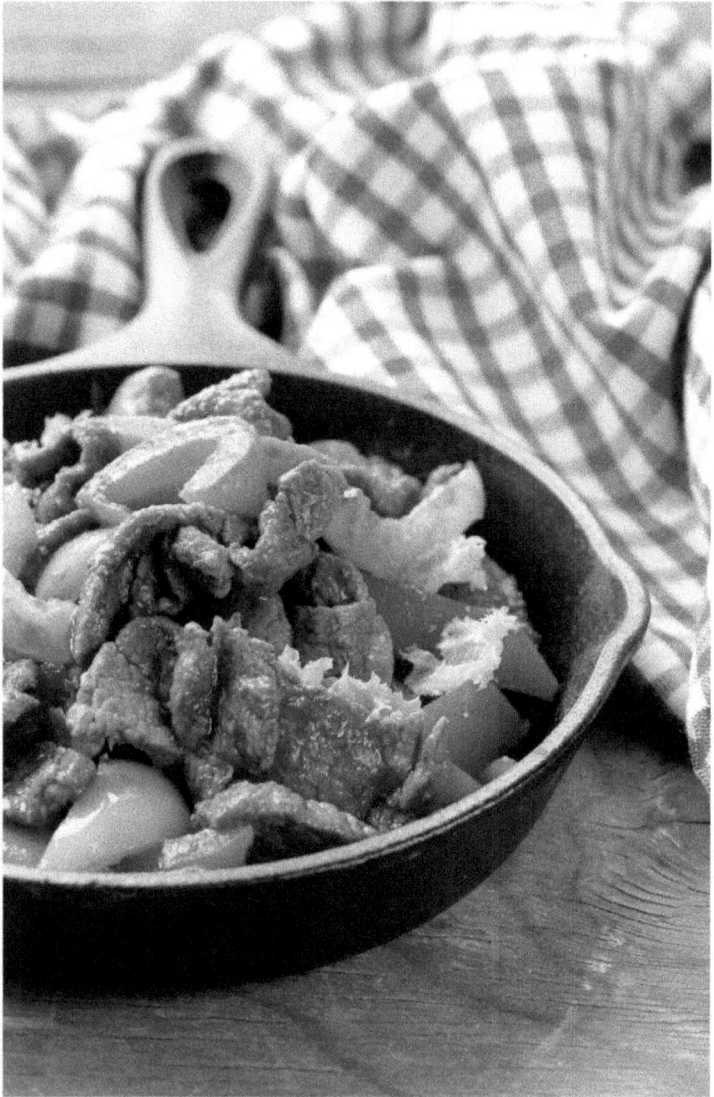

Ground Beef with Cabbage

Yield: 6 servings
Preparation Time: 10 minutes
Cooking Time: quarter-hour

Ingredients:
- 1 tbsp olive oil
- 1 onion, sliced thinly
- 2 teaspoons fresh ginger, minced
- 4 garlic cloves, minced
- 1 pound lean ground beef
- 1½ tablespoons fish sauce
- 2 tablespoons fresh lime juice
- 1 small head purple cabbage, shredded
- 2 tablespoons peanut butter
- ½ cup fresh cilantro, chopped

Directions:
1. In a large skillet, heat oil on medium heat.
2. Add onion, ginger and garlic and sauté for about 4-5 minutes.
3. Add beef and cook for approximately 7-8 minutes, getting into pieces using the spoon.
4. Drain off the extra liquid in the skillet.
5. Stir in fish sauce and lime juice and cook for approximately 1 minute.
6. Add cabbage and cook approximately 4-5 minutes or till desired doneness.
7. Stir in peanut butter and cilantro and cook for about 1 minute.
8. Serve hot.

Ground Beef with Cashews & Veggies

Yield: 4 servings

Preparation Time: 15 minutes

Cooking Time: quarter-hour

Ingredients:
- 1½ pound lean ground beef
- 1 tablespoon garlic, minced
- 2 tablespoons fresh ginger, minced
- ¼ cup coconut aminos
- Salt and freshly ground black pepper, to taste
- 1 medium onion, sliced
- 1 can water chestnuts, drained and sliced
- 1 large green bell pepper, seeded and sliced
- ½ cup raw cashews, toasted

Directions:
1. Heat a nonstick skillet on medium-high heat.

2. Add beef and cook for about 6-8 minutes breaking into pieces with the spoon.

3. Add garlic, ginger, coconut aminos, salt and black pepper and cook for approximately 2 minutes.

4. Add vegetables and cook approximately 5 minutes or till desired doneness.

5. Stir in cashews and immediately remove from heat.

6. Serve hot.

Beef & Veggies Chili

Yield: 6-8 servings
Preparation Time: 15 minutes
Cooking Time: one hour

Ingredients:
- 2 pounds lean ground beef
- ½ head cauliflower, chopped into large pieces
- 1 onion, chopped
- 6 garlic cloves, minced
- 2 cups pumpkin puree
- 1 teaspoon dried oregano, crushed
- 1 teaspoon dried thyme, crushed
- 1 teaspoon ground cumin
- 1 teaspoon ground turmeric
- 1-2 teaspoons chili powder
- 1 teaspoon paprika
- 1 teaspoon cayenne pepper
- ¼ teaspoon red pepper flakes, crushed
- Salt and freshly ground black pepper, to taste
- 1 (26-ounce) can tomatoes, drained
- ½ cup water
- 1 cup beef broth

Directions:
1. Heat a substantial pan on medium-high heat.
2. Add beef and stir fry for around 5 minutes.
3. Add cauliflower, onion and garlic and stir fry for approximately 5 minutes.

4. Add spices and herbs and stir to mix well.

5. Stir in remaining ingredients and provide to a boil.

6. Reduce heat to low and simmer, covered approximately 30-45 minutes.

7. Serve hot.

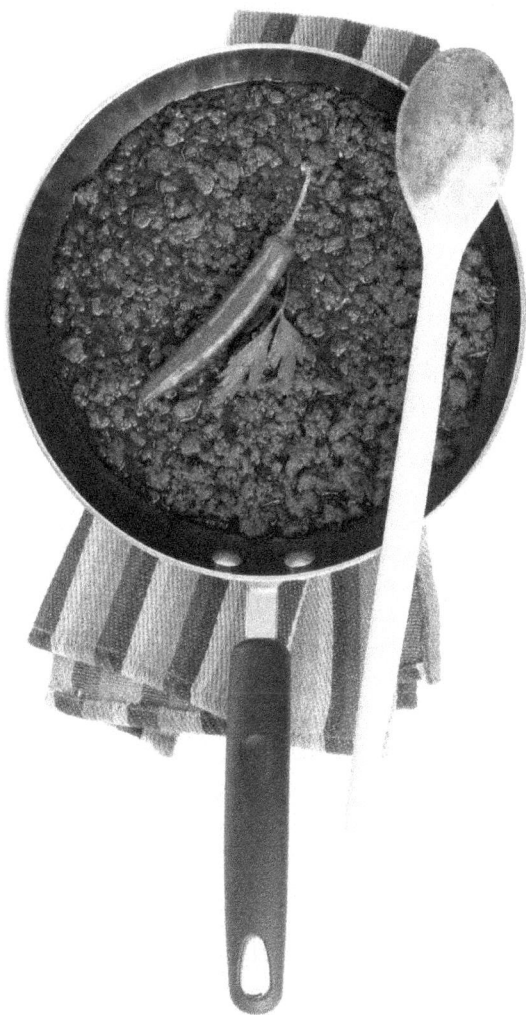

Spicy & Creamy Ground Beef Curry

Yield: 4 servings

Preparation Time: quarter-hour

Cooking Time: 32 minutes

Ingredients:

- 1-2 tablespoons coconut oil
- 1 teaspoon black mustard seeds
- 2 sprigs curry leaves
- 1 Serrano pepper, minced
- 1 large red onion, chopped finely
- 1 (1- inch) piece fresh ginger, minced
- 4 garlic cloves, minced
- 1 teaspoon ground coriander
- 1 teaspoon ground cumin
- ½ teaspoon ground turmeric
- ¼ teaspoon red chili powder
- Salt, to taste
- 1 pound lean ground beef
- 1 potato, peeled and chopped
- 3 medium carrots, peeled and chopped
- ¼ cup water
- 1 (14-ounce) can coconut milk
- Salt and freshly ground black pepper, to taste
- Chopped fresh cilantro, for garnishing

Directions:

1. In a big pan, melt coconut oil on medium heat.
2. Add mustard seeds and sauté for about thirty seconds.

3. Add curry leaves and Serrano pepper and sauté approximately half a minute.

4. Add onion, ginger and garlic and sauté for about 4-5 minutes.

5. Add spices and cook for about 1 minute.

6. Add beef and cook for about 4-5 minutes.

7. Stir in potato, carrot and water and provide with a gentle simmer.

8. Simmer, covered for around 5 minutes.

9. Stir in coconut milk and simmer for around fifteen minutes.

10. Stir in salt and black pepper and remove from heat.

11. Serve hot while using garnishing of cilantro.

Beef Meatballs in Tomato Gravy

Yield: 4 servings
Preparation Time: 20 minutes
Cooking Time: 37 minutes

Ingredients:
For Meatballs:
- 1 pound lean ground beef
- 1 organic egg, beaten
- 1 tablespoon fresh ginger, minced
- 1 garlic oil, minced
- 2 tablespoons fresh cilantro, chopped finely
- 2 tablespoons tomato paste
- 1/3 cup almond meal
- 1 tablespoon ground cumin
- Pinch of ground cinnamon
- Salt and freshly ground black pepper, to taste
- ¼ cup coconut oil

For Tomato Gravy:
- 2 tablespoons coconut oil
- ½ of small onion, chopped
- 2 garlic cloves, chopped
- 1 teaspoon fresh lemon zest, grated finely
- 2 cups tomatoes, chopped finely
- Pinch of ground cinnamon
- 1 teaspoon red pepper flakes, crushed
- ¾ cup chicken broth
- Salt and freshly ground black pepper, to taste

- ¼ cup fresh parsley, chopped

Directions:

1. For meatballs in a sizable bowl, add all ingredients except oil and mix till well combined.

2. Make about 1-inch sized balls from mixture.

3. In a substantial skillet, melt coconut oil on medium heat.

4. Add meatballs and cook for approximately 3-5 minutes or till golden brown all sides.

5. Transfer the meatballs into a bowl.

6. For gravy in a big pan, melt coconut oil on medium heat.

7. Add onion and garlic and sauté approximately 4 minutes.

8. Add lemon zest and sauté approximately 1 minute.

9. Add tomatoes, cinnamon, red pepper flakes and broth and simmer for approximately 7 minutes.

10. Stir in salt, black pepper and meatballs and reduce the warmth to medium-low.

11. Simmer for approximately twenty minutes.

12. Serve hot with all the garnishing of parsley.

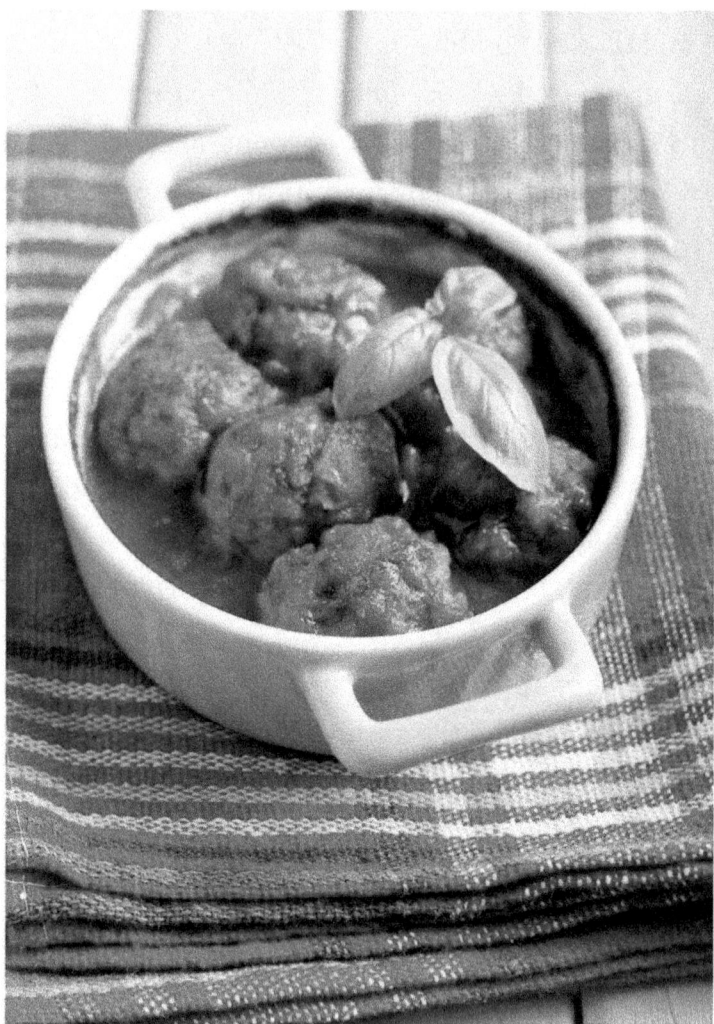

Pan Grilled Flank Steak

Yield: 3-4 servings
Preparation Time: 10 minutes
Cooking Time: 12-16 minutes

Ingredients:

- 8 medium garlic cloves, crushed
- 1 (5-inch) piece fresh ginger, sliced thinly
- 1 tablespoon organic honey
- ¼ cup organic olive oil
- Salt and freshly ground black pepper, to taste
- 1½ pound flank steak, trimmed

Directions:

1. In a large sealable bag, mix together all ingredients except steak.

2. Add steak and coat with marinade generously.

3. Seal the bag and refrigerate to marinate for approximately one day.

4. Remove from refrigerator and keep at room temperature for approximately 15 minutes.

5. Lightly, grease a grill pan as well as heat to medium-high heat.

6. Discard the surplus marinade from the steak and place in grill pan.

7. Cook for about 6-8 minutes from each party.

8. Remove from grill pan and keep aside for around 10 min before slicing.

9. With a clear, crisp knife cut into desired slices and serve.

Spicy Lamb Curry

Yield: 6-8 servings

Preparation Time: 15 minutes

Cooking Time: 2 hours quarter-hour

Ingredients:

For Spice Mixture:

- 4 teaspoons ground coriander
- 4 teaspoons ground coriander
- 4 teaspoons ground cumin
- ¾ teaspoon ground ginger
- 2 teaspoons ground cinnamon
- ½ teaspoon ground cloves
- ½ teaspoon ground cardamom
- 2 tablespoons sweet paprika
- ½ tablespoon cayenne pepper
- 2 teaspoons chili powder
- 2 teaspoons salt

For Curry:

- 1 tablespoon coconut oil
- 2 pounds boneless lamb, trimmed and cubed into 1-inch size
- Salt and freshly ground black pepper, to taste
- 2 cups onions, chopped
- 1¼ cups water
- 1 cup coconut milk

Directions:

1. For spice mixture in a bowl, mix together all spices. Keep aside.

2. Season the lamb with salt and black pepper.

3. In a large Dutch oven, heat oil on medium high heat.

4. Add lamb and stir fry for around 5 minutes.

5. Add onion and cook for approximately 4-5 minutes.

6. Stir in spice mixture and cook for approximately 1 minute.

7. Add water and coconut milk and provide to some boil on high heat.

8. Reduce the heat to low and simmer, covered for approximately 1-120 minutes or till desired doneness of lamb.

9. Uncover and simmer for approximately 3-4 minutes.

10. Serve hot.

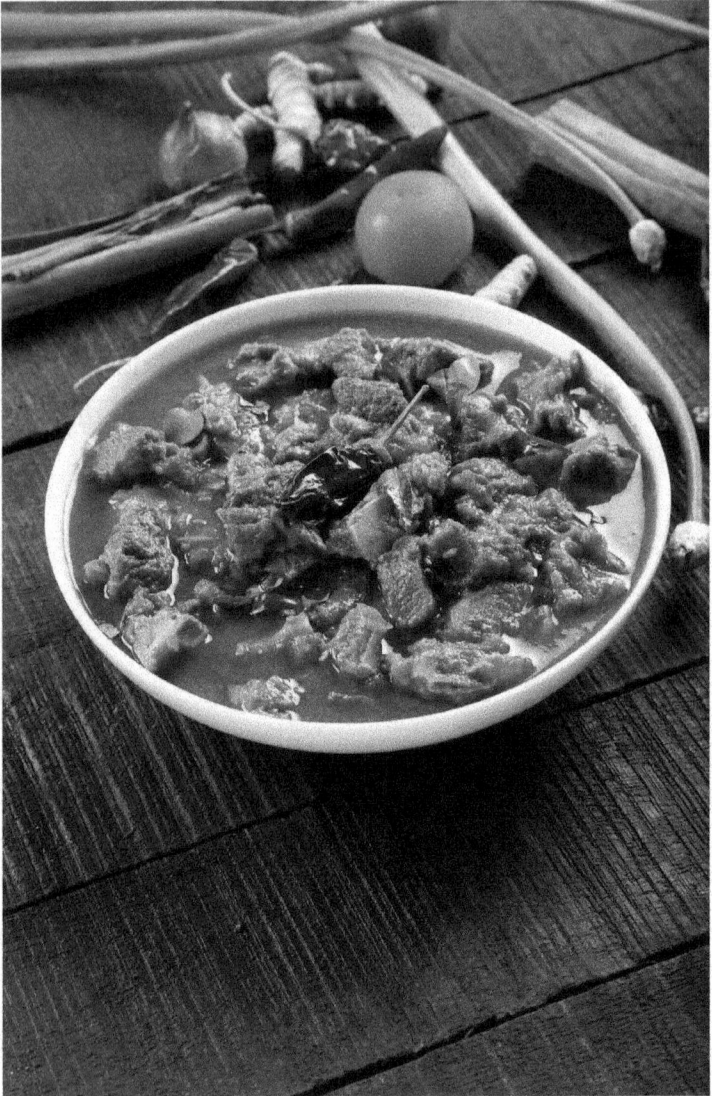

Lamb with Zucchini & Couscous

Yield: 2 servings
Preparation Time: 15 minutes
Cooking Time: 8 minutes

Ingredients:
- ¾ cup couscous
- ¾ cup boiling water
- ¼ cup fresh cilantro, chopped
- 1 tbsp olive oil
- 5-ounces lamb leg steak, cubed into ¾-inch size
- 1 medium zucchini, sliced thinly
- 1 medium red onion, cut into wedges
- 1 teaspoon ground cumin
- 1 teaspoon ground coriander
- ¼ teaspoon red pepper flakes, crushed
- Salt, to taste
- ¼ cup plain Greek yogurt
- 1 garlic herb, minced

Directions:
1. In a bowl, add couscous and boiling water and stir to combine.
2. Cover whilst aside approximately 5 minutes.
3. Add cilantro and with a fork, fluff completely.
4. Meanwhile in a substantial skillet, heat oil on high heat.
5. Add lamb and stir fry for about 2-3 minutes.
6. Add zucchini and onion and stir fry for about 2 minutes.
7. Stir in spices and stir fry for about 1 minute
8. Add couscous and stir fry approximately 2 minutes.

9. In a bowl, mix together yogurt and garlic.

10. Divide lamb mixture in serving plates evenly.

11. Serve using the topping of yogurt.

Ground Lamb with Harissa

Yield: 4 servings
Preparation Time: 15 minutes
Cooking Time: one hour 11 minutes

Ingredients:
- 1 tablespoon extra-virgin olive oil
- 2 red peppers, seeded and chopped finely
- 1 yellow onion, chopped finely
- 2 garlic cloves, chopped finely
- 1 teaspoon ground cumin
- ½ teaspoon ground turmeric
- ¼ teaspoon ground cinnamon
- ¼ teaspoon ground ginger
- 1½ pound lean ground lamb
- Salt, to taste
- 1 (14½- ounce) can diced tomatoes
- 2 tablespoons harissa
- 1 cup water
- Chopped fresh cilantro, for garnishing

Directions:
1. In a sizable pan, heat oil on medium-high heat.
2. Add bell pepper, onion and garlic and sauté for around 5 minutes.
3. Add spices and sauté for around 1 minute.
4. Add lamb and salt and cook for approximately 5 minutes, getting into pieces.
5. Stir in tomatoes, harissa and water and provide with a boil.

6. Reduce the warmth to low and simmer, covered for about 1 hour.

7. Serve hot while garnishing with harissa.

Roasted Leg of Lamb

Yield: 8 servings

Preparation Time: quarter-hour

Cooking Time: 75-100 minutes

Ingredients:

- 1/3 cup fresh parsley, minced
- 4 garlic cloves, minced
- 1 teaspoon fresh lemon zest, grated finely
- 1 tablespoon ground coriander
- 1 tablespoon ground cumin
- 1 teaspoon ground cinnamon
- 1 teaspoon ground turmeric
- 1 tablespoon sweet paprika
- ½ teaspoon allspice
- 20 saffron threads, crushed
- 1/3 cup essential olive oil
- 1 (5-pound) leg of lamb, trimmed

Directions:

1. In a bowl, mix together all ingredients except lamb.

2. Coat the leg of lamb with marinade mixture generously.

3. With a plastic wrap, cover the leg of lamb and refrigerate to marinate for about 4-8 hours. 4. Remove from refrigerator and keep at room temperature for about a half-hour before roasting.

5. Preheat the oven to 350 degrees F. Arrange the rack inside the center of the oven.

6. Lightly grease a roasting pan and make a rack inside roasting pan.

7. Place the lower limb of lamb in the rack in prepared roasting pan.

8. Roast for approximately 75-100 minutes or till desired doneness, rotating once inside the middle way.

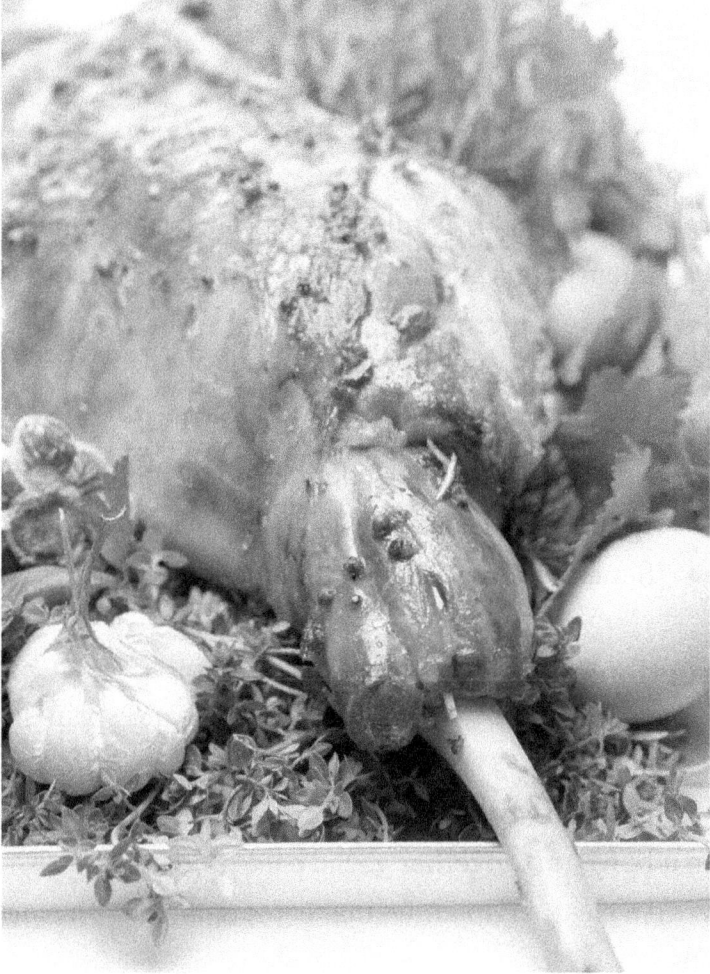

Pan-Seared Lamb Chops

Yield: 4 servings
Preparation Time: 10 minutes
Cooking Time: 4-6 minutes

Ingredients:
- 4 garlic cloves, peeled
- Salt, to taste
- 1 teaspoon black mustard seeds, crushed finely
- 2 teaspoons ground cumin
- 1 teaspoon ground ginger
- 1 teaspoon ground coriander
- ½ teaspoon ground cinnamon
- Freshly ground black pepper, to taste
- 1 tablespoon coconut oil
- 8 medium lamb chops, trimmed

Directions:
1. Place garlic cloves onto a cutting board and sprinkle with a little salt.
2. With a knife, crush the garlic till a paste forms.
3. In a bowl, mix together garlic paste and spices.
4. With a clear, crisp knife, make 3-4 cuts on both sides of the chops.
5. Rub the chops with garlic mixture generously.
6. In a large skillet, melt butter on medium heat.
7. Add chops and cook for approximately 2-3 minutes per side or till desired doneness.

Grilled Lamb Chops

Yield: 4 servings
Preparation Time: 10 min
Cooking Time: 6 minutes

Ingredients:

- 1 tablespoon fresh ginger, grated
- 4 garlic cloves, chopped roughly
- 1 teaspoon ground cumin
- ½ teaspoon red chili powder
- Salt and freshly ground black pepper, to taste
- 1 tbsp essential olive oil
- 1 tablespoon fresh lemon juice
- 8 lamb chops, trimmed

Directions:

1. In a bowl, mix together all ingredients except chops.

2. With a hand blender, blend till a smooth mixture forms.

3. Add chops and coat with mixture generously.

4. Refrigerate to marinate for overnight.

5. Preheat the barbecue grill till hot. Grease the grill grate.

6. Grill the chops for approximately 3 minutes per side.

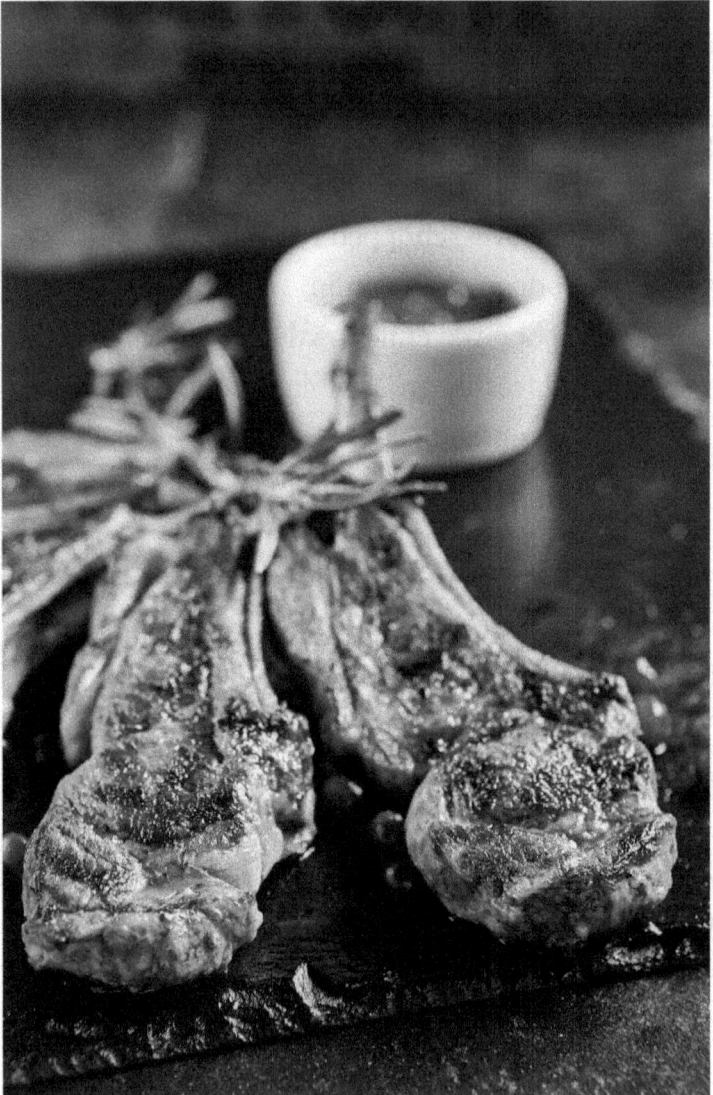

Lamb & Pineapple Kebabs

Yield: 4-6 servings
Preparation Time: 15 minutes
Cooking Time: 10 minutes

Ingredients:

- 1 large pineapple, cubed into 1½-inch size, divided
- 1 (½-inch) piece fresh ginger, chopped
- 2 garlic cloves, chopped
- Salt, to taste
- 16-24-ounce lamb shoulder steak, trimmed and cubed into 1½-inch size
- Fresh mint leaves coming from a bunch
- Ground cinnamon, to taste

Directions:

1. In a blender, add about 1½ servings of pineapple, ginger, garlic and salt and pulse till smooth.
2. Transfer the amalgamation right into a large bowl.
3. Add chops and coat with mixture generously.
4. Refrigerate to marinate for about 1-2 hours.
5. Preheat the grill to medium heat. Grease the grill grate.
6. Thread lam, remaining pineapple and mint leaves onto pre-soaked wooden skewers.
7. Grill the kebabs approximately 10 min, turning occasionally.

Fresh lime juice pork

Yield: 4 servings
Preparation Time: 15 minutes
Cooking Time: 13 minutes

Ingredients:

- 1 tablespoon fresh ginger, chopped finely
- 4 garlic cloves, chopped finely
- 1 cup fresh cilantro, chopped and divided
- ¼ cup plus 1 tbsp olive oil, divided
- 1 pound tender pork, trimmed, sliced thinly
- 2 onions, sliced thinly
- 1 green bell pepper, seeded and sliced thinly
- 1 tablespoon fresh lime juice

Directions:

1. In a substantial bowl, mix together ginger, garlic, ½ cup of cilantro and ¼ cup of oil.

2. Add pork and coat with mixture generously.

3. Refrigerate to marinate approximately a couple of hours.

4. Heat a big skillet on medium-high heat.

5. Add pork mixture and stir fry for approximately 4-5 minutes.

6. Transfer the pork right into a bowl.

7. In the same skillet, heat remaining oil on medium heat.

8. Add onion and sauté for approximately 3 minutes.

9. Stir in bell pepper and stir fry for about 3 minutes.

10. Stir in pork, lime juice and remaining cilantro and cook for about 2 minutes.

11. Serve hot.

Spiced Pork One

Yield: 6 servings
Preparation Time: fifteen minutes
Cooking Time: 60 minutes 52 minutes

Ingredients:

- 1 (2-inch) piece fresh ginger, chopped
- 5-10 garlic cloves, chopped
- 1 teaspoon ground cumin
- ½ teaspoon ground turmeric 1 tablespoon hot paprika
- 1 tablespoon red pepper flakes
- Salt, to taste
- 2 tablespoons cider vinegar
- 2 pounds pork shoulder, trimmed and cubed into 1½-inch size
- 2 cups domestic hot water, divided
- 1 (1-inch wide) ball tamarind pulp
- ¼ cup olive oil
- 1 teaspoon black mustard seeds, crushed
- 4 green cardamoms
- 5 whole cloves
- 1 (3-inch) cinnamon stick
- 1 cup onion, chopped finely
- 1 large red bell pepper, seeded and chopped

Directions:

1. In a food processor, add ginger, garlic, cumin, turmeric, paprika, red pepper flakes, salt and cider vinegar and pulse till smooth.

2. Transfer the amalgamation into a large bowl.

3. Add pork and coat with mixture generously.

4. Keep aside, covered for around an hour at room temperature.

5. In a bowl, add 1 cup of warm water and tamarind and make aside till water becomes cool. 6. With the hands, crush the tamarind to extract the pulp.

7. Add remaining cup of hot water and mix till well combined.

8. Through a fine sieve, strain the tamarind juice inside a bowl.

9. In a sizable skillet, heat oil on medium-high heat.

10. Add mustard seeds, green cardamoms, cloves and cinnamon stick and sauté for about 4 minutes.

11. Add onion and sauté for approximately 5 minutes.

12. Add pork and stir fry for approximately 6 minutes.

13. Stir in tamarind juice and convey with a boil.

14. Reduce the heat to medium-low and simmer 1½ hours.

15. Stir in bell pepper and cook for about 7 minutes.

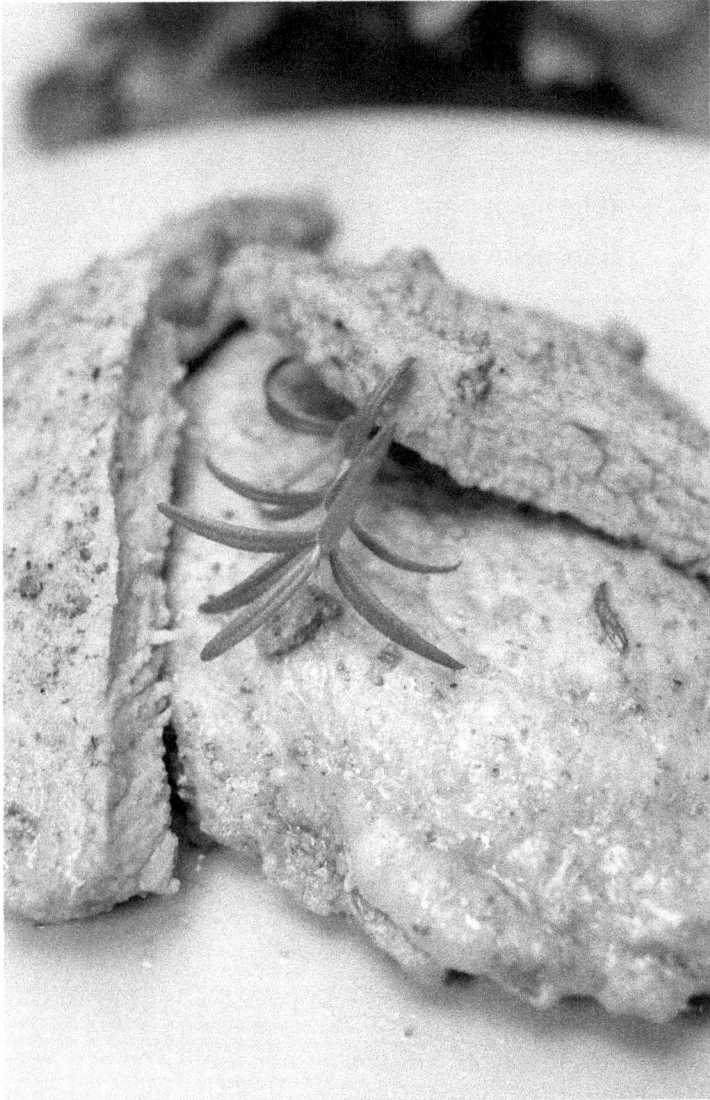

Ground Pork with Water Chestnuts

Yield: 4 servings

Preparation Time: fifteen minutes

Cooking Time: 12 minutes

Ingredients:

- 1 tablespoon plus 1 teaspoon coconut oil
- 1 tablespoon fresh ginger, minced
- 1 bunch scallion (white and green parts separated), chopped
- 1 pound lean ground pork • Salt, to taste
- 1 tablespoon 5-spice powder
- 1 (18-ounce) can water chestnuts, drained and chopped
- 1 tablespoon organic honey
- 2 tablespoons fresh lime juice

Directions:

1. In a big heavy bottomed skillet, heat oil on high heat.

2. Add ginger and scallion whites and sauté for approximately ½-1½ minutes.

3. Add pork and cook for approximately 4-5 minutes.

4. Drain the extra Fat from skillet.

5. Add salt and 5- spice powder and cook for approximately 2-3 minutes.

6. Add scallion greens and remaining ingredients and cook, stirring continuously for about 1-2 minutes.

Pork chops in Creamy Sauce

Yield: 4 servings

Preparation Time: fifteen minutes

Cooking Time: 14 minutes

Ingredients:
- 2 garlic cloves, chopped
- 1 small jalapeño pepper, chopped
- ¼ cup fresh cilantro leaves
- 1½ teaspoons ground turmeric, divided
- 1 tablespoon fish sauce
- 2 tablespoons fresh lime juice
- 1 (13½-ounce) can coconut milk
- 4 (½-inch thick) pork chops
- Salt, to taste
- 1 tablespoon coconut oil
- 1 shallot, chopped finely

Directions:

1. In a blender, add garlic, jalapeño pepper, cilantro, 1 teaspoon of ground turmeric, fish sauce, lime juice and coconut milk and pulse till smooth.

2. Sprinkle the pork with salt and remaining turmeric evenly.

3. In a skillet, melt butter on medium-high heat.

4. Add shallots and sauté approximately 1 minute.

5. Add chops and cook for approximately 2 minutes per side.

6. Transfer the chops inside a bowl.

7. Add coconut mixture and convey to your boil.

8. Reduce heat to medium and simmer, stirring occasionally for approximately 5 minutes. 9. Stir in pork chops and cook for about 3-4 minutes. 10. Serve hot.

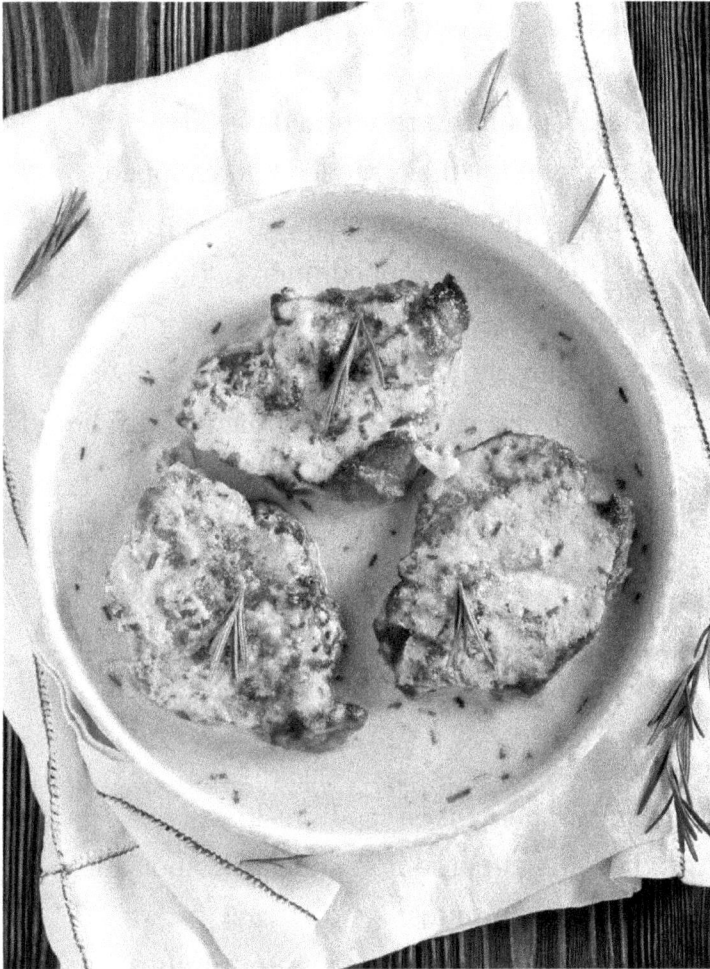

Turkey & Pumpkin Chili

Yield: 4-6 servings

Preparation Time: quarter-hour

Cooking Time: 41 minutes

Ingredients:

- 2 tablespoons extra-virgin olive oil
- 1 green bell pepper, seeded and chopped
- 1 small yellow onion, chopped
- 2 garlic cloves, chopped finely
- pound lean ground turkey
- 1 (15-ounce) pumpkin puree
- 1 (14 ½-ounce) can diced tomatoes with liquid
- 1 teaspoon ground cumin
- ½ teaspoon ground turmeric
- ½ teaspoon ground cinnamon
- 1 cup water
- 1 (15-ounce) can chickpeas, rinsed and drained

Directions:

1. In a big pan, heat oil on medium-low heat.

2. Add the bell pepper, onion and garlic and sauté approximately 5 minutes.

3. Add turkey and cook for about 5-6 minutes.

4. Add tomatoes, pumpkin, spices and water and convey to your boil on high heat.

5. Reduce the temperature to medium-low heat and stir in chickpeas.

6. Simmer, covered for approximately a half-hour, stirring occasionally.

7. Serve hot.

Ground Turkey with Lentils

Yield: 8 servings

Preparation Time: quarter-hour

Cooking Time: 35 minutes

Ingredients:

- 3 tablespoons olive oil, divided
- 1 onion, chopped
- 1 tablespoon fresh ginger, minced
- 4 garlic cloves, minced
- 2 Roma tomatoes, seeded and chopped
- 3 celery stalks, chopped
- 1 large carrot, peeled and chopped
- 1 cup dried red lentils, rinsed, soaked for thirty minutes and drained
- 2 cups chicken broth
- 1 teaspoon black mustard seeds
- 1½ teaspoons cumin seeds
- 1 teaspoon ground turmeric
- ½ teaspoon paprika
- 1 pound lean ground turkey
- 1 Serrano chile, seeded and chopped
- 2 scallions, chopped
- Chopped fresh cilantro, for garnishing

Directions:

1. In a Dutch oven, heat 1 tablespoon of oil on medium heat.
2. Add onion, ginger and garlic and sauté for around 5 minutes.

3. Stir in tomatoes, celery, carrot, lentils and broth and convey to your boil

4. Reduce the warmth to medium-low.

5. Simmer, covered for around thirty minutes.

6. Meanwhile in a skillet, heat remaining oil on medium heat.

7. Add mustard seeds and cumin seeds and sauté approximately 30 seconds.

8. Add turmeric and paprika and sauté approximately 25 seconds.

9. Transfer a combination into a small bowl and aside.

10. In exactly the same skillet, add turkey and cook for around 4-5 minutes.

11. Add Serrano chile and scallion and cook for about 3-4 minutes.

12. Add spiced oil mixture and stir to mix well.

13. Transfer the turkey mixture in simmering lentils and simmer for around 5-10 minutes more.

Grilled Turkey Breast

Yield: 4 servings
Preparation Time: 15 minutes
Cooking Time: 6-10 min

Ingredients:
- 1 large shallot, quartered
- (¾-inch) piece fresh ginger, chopped
- 2 small garlic cloves, chopped
- 1 tablespoon honey
- ¼ cup extra virgin olive oil
- ¼ cup coconut aminos
- 2 tablespoons fresh lime juice
- Freshly ground black pepper, to taste
- 4 turkey breast 10derloins

Directions:
1. In a food processor, add shallot, ginger and garlic and pulse till minced.
2. Add remaining ingredients except turkey 10derloins and pulse till well combined.
3. Transfer the mixture in a sizable bowl.
4. Add turkey 10derloins and coat with mixture generously.
5. Keep aside, covered for approximately 30 minutes.
6. Preheat the grill to medium heat. Grease the grill grate.
7. Grill for about 6-8 minutes per side.

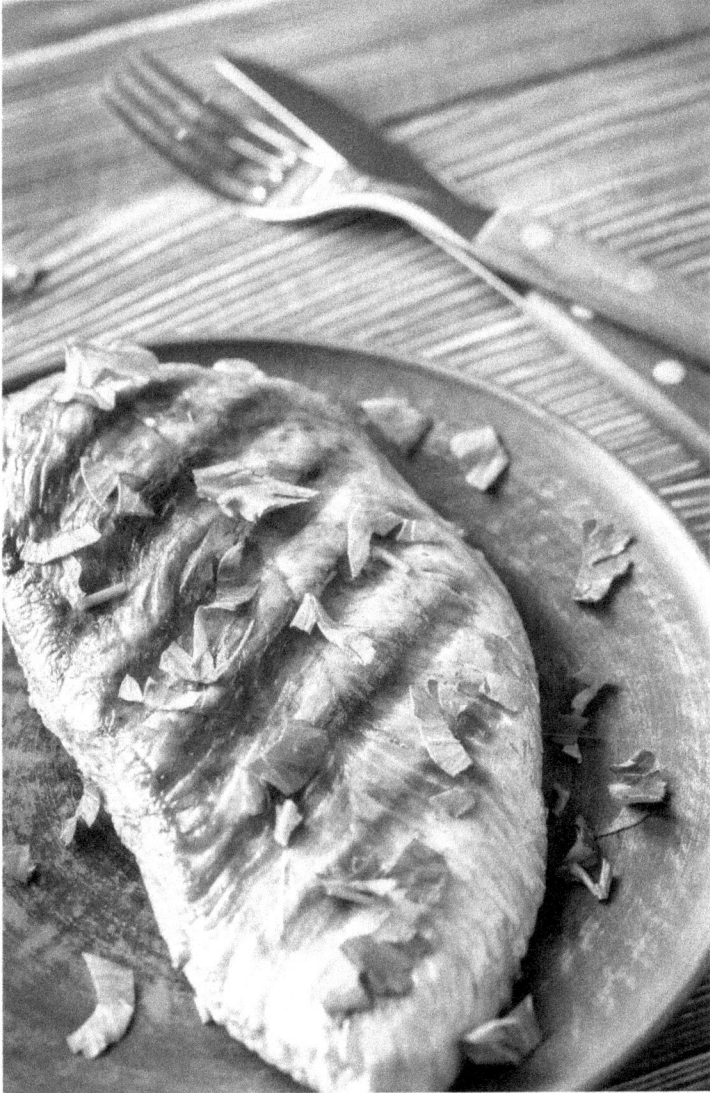

Grilled Duck Breast & Peach

Yield: 2 servings
Preparation Time: quarter-hour
Cooking Time: 24 minutes

Ingredients:
- 2 shallots, sliced thinly
- 2 tablespoons fresh ginger, minced
- 2 tablespoons fresh thyme, chopped
- Salt and freshly ground black pepper, to taste
- 2 duck breasts
- 2 peaches, pitted and quartered
- ½ teaspoon ground fennel seeds
- ½ tablespoon extra-virgin olive oil

Directions:
1. In a substantial bowl, mix together shallots, ginger, thyme, salt and black pepper.
2. Add duck breasts and coat with marinade evenly.
3. Refrigerate to marinate for about 2-12 hours.
4. Preheat the grill to medium-high heat. Grease the grill grate.
5. In a sizable bowl, add peaches, fennel seeds, salt, black pepper and oil and toss to coat well.
6. Place the duck breast on grill, skin side down and grill for around 6-8 minutes per side.
7. Transfer the duck breast onto a plate.
8. Now, grill the peaches for around 3 minutes per side.
9. Serve the duck breasts with grilled peaches.

Creamy Chicken with Broccoli & Spinach

Yield: 4 servings
Preparation Time: 15 minutes
Cooking Time: 13 minutes

Ingredients:
- 13-ounce unswee10ed coconut milk
- 1 teaspoon fresh ginger, grated
- 1½ teaspoons curry powder
- 2 tablespoons coconut oil, divided
- 1 pound 10der chicken, sliced thinly
- 1 large onion, chopped
- 2 cups broccoli florets
- 1 large bunch fresh spinach, chopped

Directions:
1. In a bowl, mix together coconut milk, ginger and curry powder. Keep aside.
2. In a big skillet, melt 1 tablespoon of coconut oil on medium-high heat.
3. Add chicken and stir fry for around 3-4 minutes or till golden brown.
4. Transfer chicken right into a plate.
5. In exactly the same skillet, heat remaining oil on medium-high heat.
6. Add onion and sauté for around 2 minutes.
7. Add broccoli and stir fry for about 3 minutes.

8. Add chicken, spinach and coconut mixture and stir fry for approximately 3-4 minutes.

Chicken with Cabbage

Yield: 4-6 servings
Preparation Time: 15 minutes
Cooking Time: 17 minutes

Ingredients:
- ½ teaspoon garlic powder
- ½ teaspoon fresh ginger powder
- Salt and freshly ground black pepper, to taste
- ½ teaspoon sesame oil
- 3 tablespoons apple cider vinegar treatment
- 4 skinless, boneless chicken breasts, sliced thinly
- 3 tablespoons coconut oil, divided
- 1 onion, sliced thinly
- 1 large head cabbage, sliced thinly
- ¼ cup organic honey
- ¼ cup coconut aminos

Directions:
1. In a big bowl, mix together garlic powder, ginger powder, salt, black pepper, sesame oil and vinegar.
2. Add chicken and coat with mixture generously whilst aside for approximately 5 minutes.
3. In a large skillet, melt 2 tablespoons of coconut oil on medium-high heat.
4. Add chicken and stir fry for about 3-4 minutes or till golden brown.
5. Transfer chicken to a plate.

6. In exactly the same skillet, melt remaining oil on medium heat.

7. Add onion and cabbage and cook for about 4-5 minutes.

8. Add chicken, honey and coconut aminos and cook for around 5-8 minutes or till desired doneness.

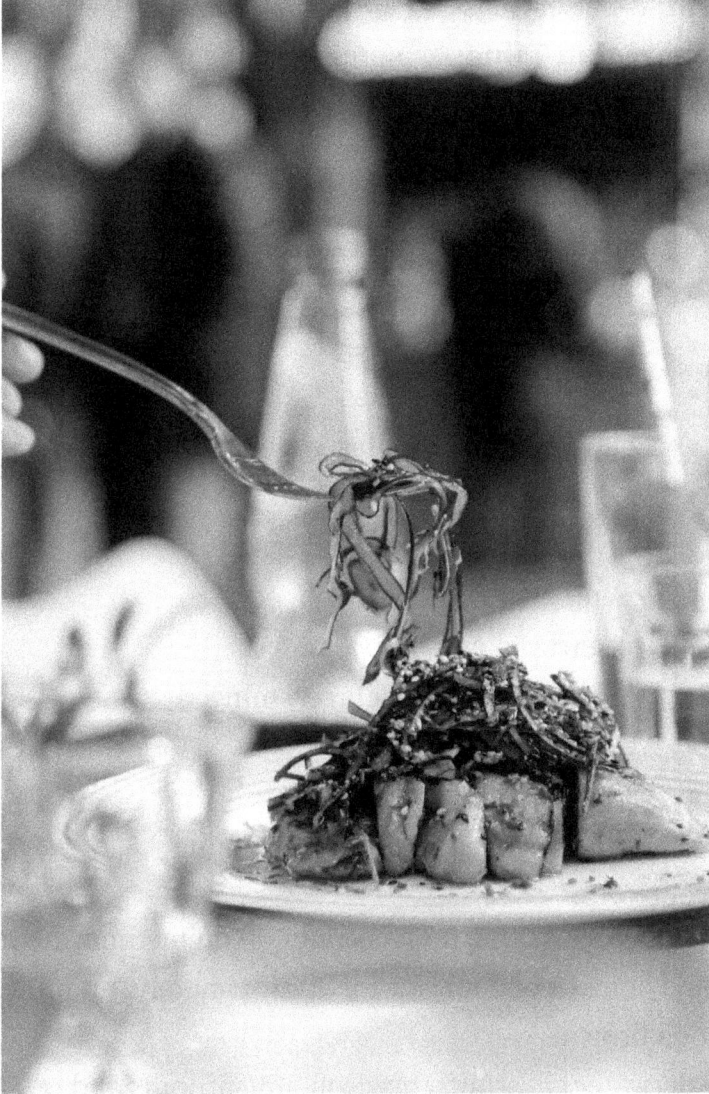

Chicken with Mixed Veggies & Almonds

Yield: 8-10 servings

Preparation Time: 25 minutes

Cooking Time: 10 min

Ingredients:

- 2 tablespoons coconut oil
- 2 skinless, boneless chicken breasts, cubed
- 2 (8- ounce) cans water chestnuts
- 4 cups broccoli florets
- 1 cup fresh mushrooms, sliced
- ½ cup celery stalk, chopped
- 1 head cabbage, shredded
- ½ cup green onions, chopped
- 4-5 garlic cloves, minced
- 2 tablespoons fresh ginger, minced
- ½ cup almonds, chopped
- 3 tablespoons coconut aminos
- White sesame seeds, for garnishing

Directions:

1. In a sizable skillet, melt coconut oil on medium-high heat.

2. Add chicken and stir fry for approximately 3-4 minutes or till golden brown.

3. Add water chestnuts, broccoli, mushrooms and celery and stir fry for around 2 minutes.

4. Add cabbage, green onion, garlic, ginger, almonds and coconut aminos and cook for approximately 2-3 minutes.

5. Serve hot with the garnishing of sesame seeds.

Chicken with Strawberries, Rhubarb & Zucchini

Yield: 2 servings
Preparation Time: twenty or so minutes
Cooking Time: 13 minutes

Ingredients:
- 2 zucchinis, spiralized with Blade C
- Salt, to taste • 1½ teaspoons olive oil
- ½ teaspoon fresh ginger, minced
- ¾ cup rhubarb, chopped
- 1 (8-ounce) skinless, boneless chicken breasts, cubed
- 4 teaspoons organic honey
- 1 teaspoon fresh lime zest, grated finely
- ¼ cup plus 2 teaspoons fresh orange juice, divided
- 1 tablespoon fresh lime juice
- 2 teaspoons fresh mint leaves, minced
- ½ cup fresh strawberries, hulled and sliced
- 2 tablespoons almonds, toasted and slivered

Directions:
1. Arrange a sizable strainer over sink.
2. Place the zucchini noodles in strainer and sprinkle using a pinch of salt.
3. Keep aside and release the moisture.
4. In a sizable skillet, heat oil on medium heat.

5. Add ginger and rhubarb and cook for about 2-3 minutes.

6. Stir in chicken and cook for approximately 4-5 minutes.

7. Add honey, lime zest, ¼ cup of orange juice, lime juice and pinch of salt and cook and raise the heat to high.

8. Bring to your boil reducing heat to medium.

9. Simmer, stirring occasionally approximately 4-5 minutes and take off from heat.

10. Squeeze the moisture from zucchini and pat dry with paper towels.

11. In a smaller bowl, mix together remaining orange juice and mint.

12. Divide zucchini noodles in serving plates and drizzle with mint mixture.

13. Place chicken mixture, strawberries and almonds over zucchini noodles and gently stir to combine.

14. Serve immediately.

Lemon Braised Chicken

Yield: 6 servings
Preparation Time: fifteen minutes
Cooking Time: one hour

Ingredients:
- 2 tablespoons organic olive oil
- 6 bone-in chicken thighs
- Salt and freshly ground black pepper, to taste
- ½ of onion, sliced
- 4 cups chicken broth
- 8 sprigs fresh dill
- Pinch of cayenne pepper
- ½ teaspoon ground turmeric
- 2 tablespoons fresh lemon juice
- 2 tablespoons arrowroot starch
- 1 tablespoon cold water
- ½ tablespoon fresh dill, chopped

Directions:
1. In a substantial skillet, heat oil on high heat.
2. Sprinkle the chicken with salt and black pepper.
3. Place inside the skillet, skin side down and cook for about 3-4 minutes.
4. Transfer the thighs in a very plate.
5. In a similar skillet, add onion on medium heat and sauté approximately 4-5 minutes.
6. Return the thighs in the skillet, skin side up with broth.

7. Place the dill sprigs over thighs and sprinkle with cayenne, turmeric and salt.

8. Bring to some boil reducing the warmth to medium-low.

9. Simmer, covered for around 40-45 minutes, coating the thighs with cooking liquid.

10. Meanwhile in a small bowl, mix together arrowroot starch and water.

11. Discard the thyme sprigs and transfer the thighs into a bowl.

12. Stir in freshly squeezed lemon juice in sauce.

13. Slowly, add arrowroot starch mixture, stirring continuously.

14. Cook, stirring occasionally for approximately 3-4 minutes or till desired thickness.

15. Serve hot using the topping of chopped dill.

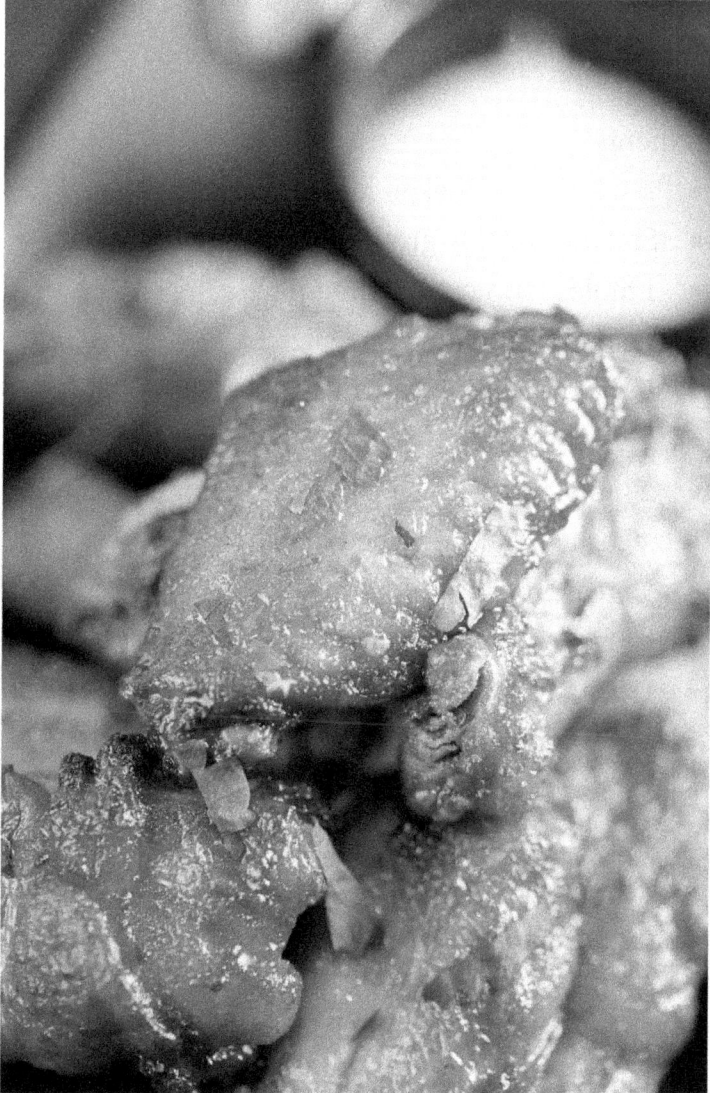

Herbed Chicken with Olives

Yield: 4 servings

Preparation Time: fifteen minutes

Cooking Time: 60 minutes 45 minutes

Ingredients:

- 4-6 bone-in chicken legs and thighs
- Salt and freshly ground black pepper, to taste
- 1 tablespoon fresh lemon juice
- 1 cup olives, pitted and sliced
- ¼ cup essential olive oil
- 2 medium yellow onions, sliced thinly
- 2 tablespoons fresh lemon zest, grated finely
- 3 garlic cloves, crushed
- ½ teaspoon ground ginger
- ¼ teaspoon saffron threads, crushed
- 1½ cups chicken broth
- ¼ cup fresh parsley leaves, chopped
- ¼ cup fresh cilantro leaves, chopped

Directions:

1. Drizzle the chicken with all the freshly squeezed lemon juice and sprinkle with salt and black pepper.

2. In a substantial Dutch oven, heat oil on medium high heat.

3. Add chicken and cook for around 4-6 minutes per side.

4. Add remaining ingredients except herbs and bring to a boil.

5. Reduce the heat to medium-low.

6. Simmer for around 75 minutes.

7. Stir in herbs and simmer for quarter-hour more.

8. Serve immediately.

Chicken Chili with Zucchini

Yield: 4-5 servings
Preparation Time: 15 minutes
Cooking Time: 35 minutes

Ingredients:

- 3 tablespoons organic olive oil
- 1 poblano pepper, seeded and chopped
- ½ of red onion, chopped
- 1 tablespoon garlic, minced
- 1 zucchini, halved lengthwise and sliced
- 2 (15-ounce) cans cannellini beans, rinsed and drained
- 1½ cups rotisserie chicken, shredded
- 1 tablespoon fresh oregano, minced
- 1 teaspoon ground turmeric
- 1 teaspoon ground cumin
- Salt and freshly ground black pepper, to taste
- 2 cups water
- 2 cups chicken broth
- 1/3 cup sharp cheddar cheese, shredded
- Chopped chives, for garnishing

Directions:

1. In a substantial pan, heat oil on medium-low heat.

2. Add poblano pepper and onion and sauté for approximately 10 min.

3. Add garlic and zucchini and cook for around 5 minutes.

4. Add remaining ingredients except cheese and chives and produce to your boil.

5. Reduce the heat to low and simmer for around twenty minutes.

6. Add the cheese and stir till well combined.

7. Serve hot with the topping of chives.

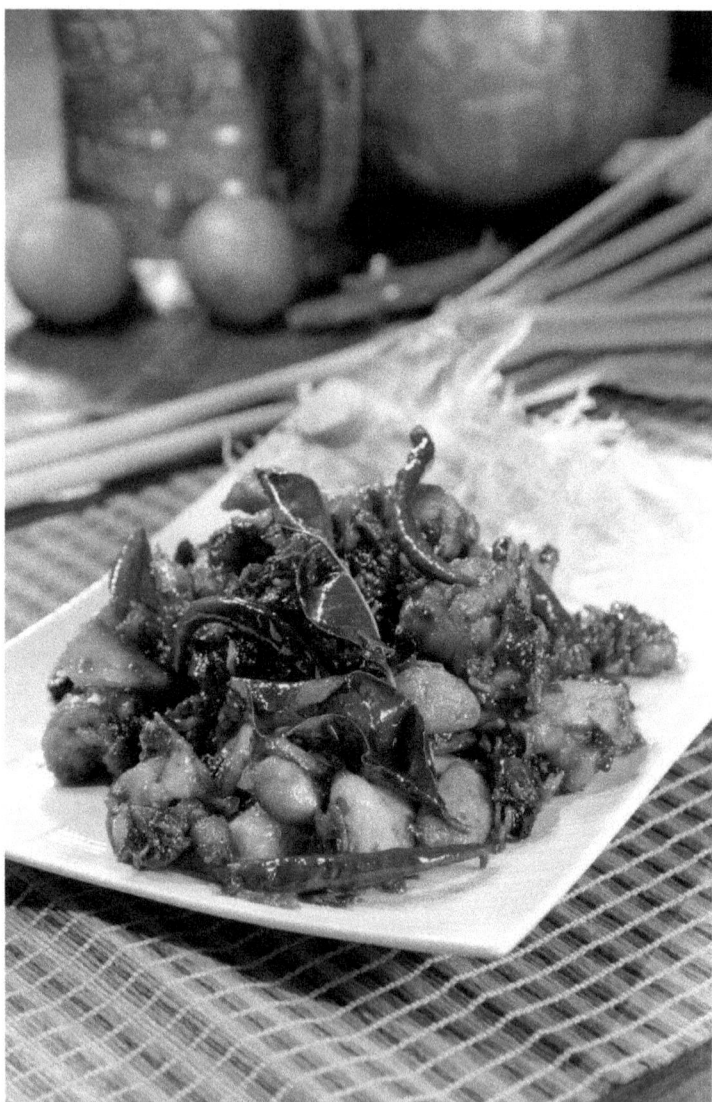

Chicken Chili with Two Beans & Corn

Yield: 6 servings
Preparation Time: quarter-hour
Cooking Time: 28 minutes

Ingredients:
- 1 tbsp essential olive oil
- 1 pound skinless, boneless chicken, cubed into 1-inch size
- 1 cup onion, chopped
- 1 cup green bell pepper, seeded and chopped
- 1½ teaspoons dried oregano, crushed
- 1 teaspoon garlic powder
- 1 teaspoon ground cumin
- 1 tablespoon paprika
- ¼ teaspoon red pepper flakes, crushed
- 1 cup frozen corn
- 1 (14½-ounce) can diced tomatoes with liquid
- 1 (15-ounce) can great Northern beans, rinsed and drained
- 1 (15-ounce) can black beans, rinsed and drained
- 1 cup chicken broth

Directions:
1. In a substantial pan, heat oil on medium-high heat.

2. Add chicken, onion and bell pepper and sauté approximately 6-8 minutes.

3. Add oregano and spices and stir to blend well.

4. Add remaining ingredients and provide to your boil.

5. Reduce the temperature to low and simmer for about twenty minutes.

6. Serve hot.

Chicken & Sweet Potato Curry

Yield: 4 servings
Preparation Time: fifteen minutes
Cooking Time: 6-10 minutes

Ingredients:

- 2 tablespoons organic olive oil, divided
- Salt and freshly ground black pepper, to taste
- 1 pound skinless, boneless chicken breast, cut into chunks
- ½ of onion, chopped
- 2 minced garlic cloves
- 1 teaspoon ground ginger
- 1 teaspoon curry powder
- ½ cup chicken broth
- 2 large sweet potatoes, peeled and cubed
- 1 can coconut milk

Directions:

1. In a sizable skillet, heat 1 tablespoon of oil on medium heat.

2. Add chicken and sprinkle with salt and black pepper.

3. Stir fry approximately 3-4 minutes per side.

4. Transfer chicken right into a plate.

5. In the identical skillet, heat remaining oil on medium heat.

6. Add onion and sauté for about 5-7 minutes.

7. Add garlic, ground ginger and curry powder and sauté for around 1-2 minutes.

8. Add chicken and remaining ingredients and stir to mix well.

9. Simmer, covered for around 15-twenty minutes.

10. Stir in salt and black pepper and serve hot.

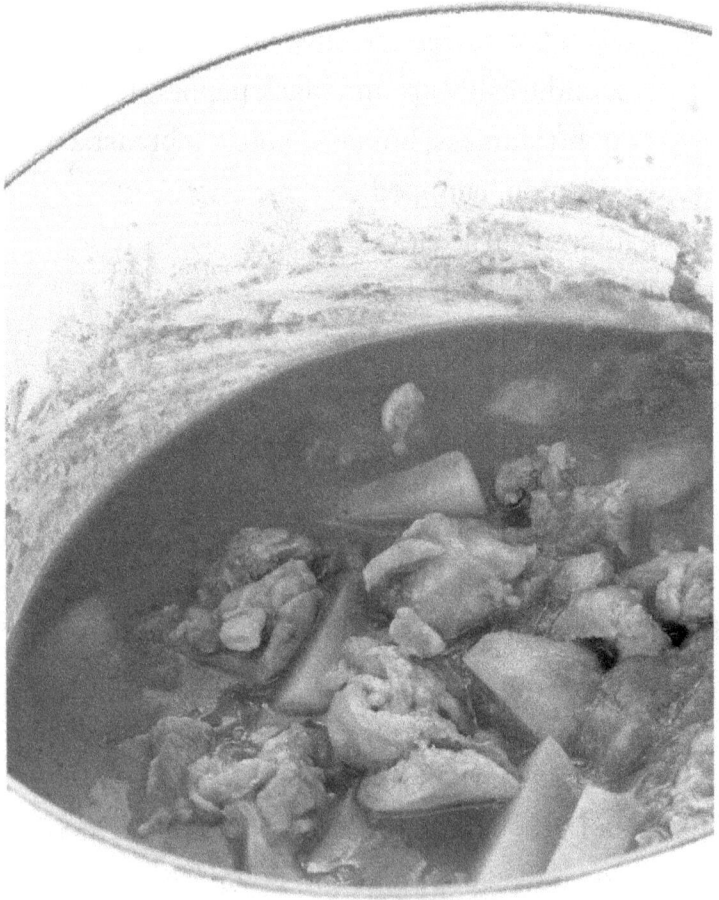

Chicken Meatballs Curry

Yield: 3-4 servings
Preparation Time: 20 min
Cooking Time: 25 minutes

Ingredients:
For Meatballs:

- 1 pound lean ground chicken
- 1 tablespoon onion paste
- 1 teaspoons fresh ginger paste
- 1 teaspoons garlic paste
- 1 green chili, chopped finely
- 1 tablespoon fresh cilantro leaves, chopped
- 1 teaspoon ground coriander
- ½ teaspoon cumin seeds
- ½ teaspoon red chili powder
- ½ teaspoon ground turmeric
- Salt, to taste

For Curry:

- 3 tablespoons extra-virgin olive oil
- ½ teaspoon cumin seeds
- 1 (1-inch) cinnamon stick
- 3 whole cloves • 3 whole green cardamoms
- 1 whole black cardamom
- 2 onions, chopped
- 1 teaspoons fresh ginger, minced
- 1 teaspoons garlic, minced
- 4 whole tomatoes, chopped finely

- 2 teaspoons ground coriander
- 1 teaspoon garam masala powder
- ½ teaspoon ground nutmeg
- ½ teaspoon red chili powder
- ½ teaspoon ground turmeric
- Salt, to taste
- 1 cup water
- Chopped fresh cilantro, for garnishing

Directions:
1. For meatballs in a substantial bowl, add all ingredients and mix till well combined.
2. Make small equal-sized meatballs from mixture.
3. In a big deep skillet, heat oil on medium heat.
4. Add meatballs and fry approximately 3-5 minutes or till browned from all sides.
5. Transfer the meatballs in a bowl.
6. In the same skillet, add cumin seeds, cinnamon stick, cloves, green cardamom and black cardamom and sauté approximately 1 minute.
7. Add onions and sauté for around 4-5 minutes.
8. Add ginger and garlic paste and sauté approximately 1 minute.
9. Add tomato and spices and cook, crushing with the back of a spoon for approximately 2-3 minutes.
10. Add water and meatballs and provide to a boil.
11. Reduce heat to low.
12. Simmer for approximately 10 minutes.
13. Serve hot with all the garnishing of cilantro.

Chicken & Veggie Casserole

Yield: 4 servings
Preparation Time: quarter-hour
Cooking Time: half an hour

Ingredients:
- 1/3 cup Dijon mustard
- 1/3 cup organic honey
- 1 teaspoon dried basil
- ¼ teaspoon ground turmeric
- 1 teaspoon dried basil, crushed
- Salt and freshly ground black pepper, to taste
- 1¾ pound chicken breasts
- 1 cup fresh white mushrooms, sliced
- ½ head broccoli, cut into small florets

Directions:
1. Preheat the oven to 350 degrees F. Lightly, grease a baking dish.
2. In a bowl, mix together all ingredients except chicken, mushrooms and broccoli.
3. Arrange chicken in the prepared baking dish and top with mushroom slices.
4. Place broccoli florets around chicken evenly.
5. Pour 1 / 2 of honey mixture over chicken and broccoli evenly.
6. Bake for approximately twenty minutes.
7. Now, coat the chicken with remaining sauce and bake for approximately 10 minutes.

Chicken Meatloaf with Veggies

Yield: 4 servings
Preparation Time: 20 minutes
Cooking Time: 1-1¼ hours

Ingredients:
For Meatloaf:

- ½ cup cooked chickpeas
- 2 egg whites
- 2½ teaspoons poultry seasoning
- Salt and freshly ground black pepper, to taste
- 10-ounce lean ground chicken
- 1 cup red bell pepper, seeded and minced
- 1 cup celery stalk, minced
- 1/3 cup steel-cut oats
- 1 cup tomato puree, divided
- 2 tablespoons dried onion flakes, crushed
- 1 tablespoon prepared mustard

For Veggies:

- 2 pounds summer squash, sliced
- 16-ounce frozen Brussels sprouts
- 2 tablespoons extra virgin extra virgin olive oil
- Salt and freshly ground black pepper, to taste

Directions:
1. Preheat the oven to 350 degrees F. Grease a 9x5-inch loaf pan.
2. In a mixer, add chickpeas, egg whites, poultry seasoning, salt and black pepper and pulse till smooth.

3. Transfer a combination in a large bowl.

4. Add chicken, veggies oats, ½ cup of tomato puree and onion flakes and mix till well combined.

5. Transfer the amalgamation into prepared loaf pan evenly.

6. With both hands, press down the amalgamation slightly.

7. In another bowl mix together mustard and remaining tomato puree.

8. Place the mustard mixture over the loaf pan evenly.

9. Bake approximately 1-1¼ hours or till desired doneness.

10. Meanwhile in a big pan of water, arrange a steamer basket.

11. Bring to a boil and set squash in the steamer basket.

12. Cover and steam approximately 10-12 minutes.

13. Drain well and aside.

14. Now, prepare the Brussels sprouts according to package's directions.

15. In a big bowl, add veggies, oil, salt and black pepper and toss to coat well.

16. Serve the meatloaf with veggies.

Roasted Chicken with Veggies & Orange

Yield: 4 servings
Preparation Time: 20 min
Cooking Time: 60 minutes

Ingredients:

- 1 teaspoon ground ginger
- ½ teaspoon ground cumin
- ½ teaspoon ground coriander
- 1 teaspoon paprika
- Salt and freshly ground black pepper, to taste
- 1 (3 ½-4-pound) whole chicken
- 1 unpeeled orange, cut into 8 wedges
- 2 medium carrots, peeled and cut into 2-inch pieces
- 2 medium sweet potatoes, peeled and cut into ½-inch wedges
- ½ cup water

Directions:

1. Preheat the oven to 450 degrees F.
2. In a little bowl, mix together the spices.
3. Rub the chicken with spice mixture evenly.
4. Arrange the chicken in a substantial Dutch oven and put orange, carrot and sweet potato pieces around it.
5. Add water and cover the pan tightly.
6. Roast for around 30 minutes.
7. Uncover and roast for about half an hour.

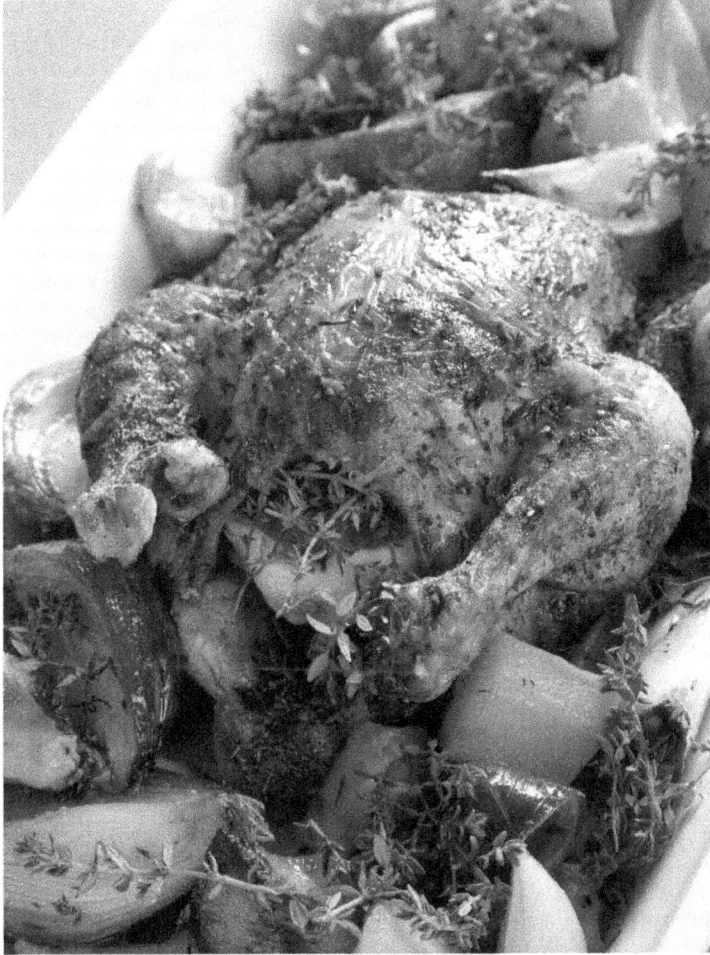

Roasted Chicken Drumsticks

Yield: 4-6 servings
Preparation Time: fifteen minutes
Cooking Time: 50 minutes

Ingredients:
- 1 medium onion, chopped
- 1-2 tablespoons fresh turmeric, chopped
- 1-2 tablespoons fresh ginger, chopped
- 2 lemongrass stalks (bottom third), peeled and chopped
- 1-2 jalapeños, seeded and chopped
- 1 teaspoon fresh lime zest, grated
- 1 tablespoon curry powder
- 1¼ cups unswee1oed coconut milk
- 3 tablespoons fresh lime juice
- 1 tablespoon coconut aminos
- 1 tablespoon fish sauce
- 3-4 pound chicken legs
- Chopped fresh cilantro, for garnishing

Directions:
1. In a blender, add all ingredients except chicken legs and pulse till smooth.

2. Transfer a combination in a large baking dish.

3. Add chicken and coat with marinade generously.

4. Cover and refrigerate to marinade approximately 12 hours.

5. Remove chicken from refrigerator and keep at room temperature approximately 25-half an hour before cooking.

6. Preheat the oven to 350 degrees F.

7. Uncover the baking dish and roast for about 50 minutes.

Grilled Chicken Breast

Yield: 4 servings
Preparation Time: 15 minutes
Cooking Time: 20 minutes

Ingredients:
- 2 scallions, chopped
- 1 (1-inch) piece fresh ginger, minced
- 2 minced garlic cloves
- 1 cup fresh pineapple juice
- ¼ cup coconut aminos
- ¼ cup extra-virgin organic olive oil
- 1 teaspoon ground cinnamon
- 1 teaspoon ground cumin
- 1 teaspoon ground turmeric
- Salt, to taste
- 4 skinless, boneless chicken breasts

Directions:
1. In a big ziploc bag add all ingredients and seal it.
2. Shake the bag to coat the chicken with marinade well.
3. Refrigerate to marinade for about twenty or so minutes to an hour.
4. Preheat the grill to medium-high heat. Grease the grill grate.
5. Place the chicken pieces on grill and grill for about 10 min per side.

Ground Turkey with Veggies

Yield: 4 servings

Preparation Time: quarter-hour

Cooking Time: 12 minutes

Ingredients:
- 1 tablespoon sesame oil
- 1 tablespoon coconut oil
- 1 pound lean ground turkey
- 2 tablespoons fresh ginger, minced
- 2 minced garlic cloves
- 1 (16-ounce) bag vegetable mix (broccoli, carrot, cabbage, kale and Brussels sprouts)
- ¼ cup coconut aminos
- 2 tablespoons balsamic vinegar

Directions:
1. In a big skillet, heat both oils on medium-high heat.
2. Add turkey, ginger and garlic and cook for approximately 5-6 minutes.
3. Add vegetable mix and cook for approximately 4-5 minutes.
4. Stir in coconut aminos and vinegar and cook for about 1 minute.
5. Serve hot.

Ground Turkey with Peas & Potato

Yield: 4 servings
Preparation Time: fifteen minutes
Cooking Time: 35 minutes

Ingredients:

- 3-4 tablespoons coconut oil
- 1 pound lean ground turkey
- 1-2 fresh red chiles, chopped
- 1 onion, chopped
- Salt, to taste
- 2 minced garlic cloves
- 1 (1-inch) piece fresh ginger, grated finely
- 1 tablespoon curry powder
- 1 teaspoon ground coriander
- 1 teaspoon ground cumin
- 1 teaspoon ground turmeric
- 2 large Yukon gold potatoes, peeled and cubed into 1-inch size
- ½ cup water
- 1 cup fresh peas, shelled
- 2-4 plum tomatoes, chopped
- ½ cup fresh cilantro, chopped

Directions:

1. In a substantial pan, heat oil on medium-high heat.
2. Add turkey and cook for about 4-5 minutes.
3. Add chiles and onion and cook for about 4-5 minutes.
4. Add garlic and ginger and cook approximately 1-2 minutes.

5. Stir in spices, potatoes and water and convey to your boil

6. Reduce the warmth to medium-low.

7. Simmer, covered approximately 15-twenty or so minutes.

8. Add peas and tomatoes and cook for about 2-3 minutes.

9. Serve using the garnishing of cilantro.

Notes

www.ingramcontent.com/pod-product-compliance
Lightning Source LLC
Chambersburg PA
CBHW050757030426
42336CB00012B/1856